1. SUBJECT AREA: Innate immunity
QUESTION: Which of the follo surfaces:

A: Skin
B: Mucus
C: Gastric acid
D: Salivary amylase
E: Gut microflora

☐ Correct Answer: D

Learning Response A: Incorrect. Intact skin prevents entry of microorganisms. Damage as in burns causes vulnerability to infection.

Learning Response B: Incorrect. Mucus lining the mucosal surfaces of the body tends to inhibit direct attachment of infectious microorganisms to the mucosal surface.

Learning Response C: Incorrect. Gastric acid provides a hostile environment to many microorganisms.

Learning Response D: Correct. The enzyme splits starch and is of importance for digestion but not for protection.

Learning Response E: Incorrect. Gut microflora produce antibiotic substances, colicins, which can kill other bacteria.

2. SUBJECT AREA: Phagocytosis
QUESTION: The mononuclear phagocyte system does not include:

A: Monocytes
B: Kupffer cells
C: Kidney mesangial cells
D: Lymph node medullary macrophages
E: Endothelial cells

☐ Correct Answer: E

Learning Response A: Incorrect. Monocytes circulate in the blood being derived from hemopoietic myeloid stem cells.

Learning Response B: Incorrect. Monocytes settle to become phagocytic cells in the liver.

Learning Response C: Incorrect. The mononuclear phagocytes which form the mesangium in the glomeruli are part of this system.

Learning Response D: Incorrect. Macrophages lining the medullary sinuses are part of the mononuclear phagocyte system.

Learning Response E: Correct. Endothelial cells are not essentially phagocytic although they do contribute, by the production of mediators, to the inflammatory process, particularly the acute inflammatory process. They were previously lumped together with the mononuclear phagocyte system in what was known as the reticuloendothelial system (RES).

---

3. SUBJECT AREA: Phagocytosis
QUESTION: A polymorphonuclear neutrophil:

- *A:* Is a bone marrow stem cell
- *B:* Is closely similar to a mast cell
- *C:* Contains microbicidal cytoplasmic granules
- *D:* Is not a "professional" phagocytic cell
- *E:* Has granules which stain with eosin

☐ Correct Answer: *C*

Learning Response A: Incorrect. The bone marrow stem cell is the precursor of the formed elements of the blood which include the PMN.

Learning Response B: Incorrect. The granular polymorphonuclear cell that stains with basic dyes, i.e., the basophil, is similar to a mast cell.

Learning Response C: Correct. The granules contain a wide spectrum of microbicidal agents.

Learning Response D: Incorrect. The major professional phagocytic cells are the polymorphs and the macrophages.

Learning Response E: Incorrect. The word neutrophil implies the granules stain neither with acid nor basic dyes. The eosinophil has granules that stain with the acid dye and are important in defense against parasitic infections.

4. SUBJECT AREA: Phagocytosis
QUESTION: Bacteria can be damaged by reactive oxygen intermediates such as:

$A:$ $O_2^-\cdot$
$B:$ O_2
$C:$ OH^-
$D:$ NO
$E:$ NO_2

☐ Correct Answer: A

Learning Response A: Correct. This is the superoxide anion obtained by addition of an electron to molecular oxygen by the cytochrome P-245 oxidase system.

Learning Response B: Incorrect. Oxygen is not a reactive intermediate.

Learning Response C: Incorrect. The hydroxyl ion has no effect.

Learning Response D: Incorrect. Nitric oxide is a powerful antimicrobicidal agent but it is *not* a reactive *oxygen* intermediate.

Learning Response E: Incorrect. Nitrogen peroxide is not formed in any appreciable amounts in the body and is not bactericidal.

---

5. SUBJECT AREA: Phagocytosis
QUESTION: Polymorph defensins are:

$A:$ Antitoxins
$B:$ Oxygen-dependent
$C:$ Enzymes
$D:$ Cationic proteins
$E:$ Peptide antibiotics

☐ Correct Answer: E

Learning Response A: Incorrect. Antitoxins are usually antibodies.

Learning Response B: Incorrect. The defensins are part of the oxygen-independent defensive system of the polymorph.

Learning Response C: Incorrect. There are enzymes within the polymorph granules, some of which participate in the production of reactive intermediates and some which help the digestion of killed microorganisms.

Learning Response D: Incorrect. The cationic proteins are granule components which are antimicrobial.

Learning Response *E:* Correct. The peptides present in the granules are in extremely high concentration.

---

6. SUBJECT AREA: Complement
QUESTION: Complement component C3 is cleaved by:

A: C3b
B: C3bBb
C: Factor B
D: Factor D
E: Factor H

☐ Correct Answer: *B*

Learning Response A: Incorrect. C3b is an opsonizing agent that assists phagocytosis and also contributes to some of the cleavage enzymes.

Learning Response B: Correct. This is the C3 convertase enzyme generated in the alternative complement pathway and is responsible for splitting off the small peptide C3a leaving C3b as a residue.

Learning Response C: Incorrect. Factor B contributes to the alternative pathway C3 convertase. See learning response B.

Learning Response D: Incorrect. Factor D splits Factor B to form Bb.

Learning Response E: Incorrect. Factor H combines with C3b making it vulnerable to cleavage by Factor I. It displaces Factor Bb from the convertase so leading to its destabilization.

---

7. SUBJECT AREA: Complement
QUESTION: The membrane attack complex consists of:

A: OH
B: Colicins

C: C3b, 3b, Bb
D: C5b, 6, 7, 8, 9
E: Properdin

☐ Correct Answer: *D*

Learning Response A: Incorrect. The hydroxyl radical is a reactive oxygen intermediate.

Learning Response B: Incorrect. The colicins are antibiotics produced by the gut microflora.

Learning Response C: Incorrect. This is the convertase which splits component C5 to give C5a and C5b.

Learning Response D: Correct. These terminal components form a complex which inserts into the membrane to form a transmembrane ion channel which lyses the cell.

Learning Response E: Incorrect. Properdin is a component of the alternative pathway which stabilizes the C3bBb C3 convertase.

8. SUBJECT AREA: Complement
QUESTION: C3b:

A: Is chemotactic
B: Is an anaphylatoxin
C: Opsonizes bacteria
D: Directly injures bacteria
E: Is the inactive form of C3

☐ Correct Answer: *C*

Learning Response A: Incorrect. C5a is chemotactic.

Learning Response B: Incorrect. C3a, a small peptide split off from the parent C3 molecule, is an anaphylatoxin like C5a and degranulates mast cells.

Learning Response C: Correct. The bacteria coated with C3b adhere to C3b receptors on professional phagocytic cells.

Learning Response D: Incorrect. There is no evidence for this.

Learning Response E: Incorrect. The inactive form of C3 is obtained by splitting the C3b to form iC3b, C3d and C3de.

---

9. SUBJECT AREA: Inflammation
QUESTION: Acute inflammation characteristically involves:

A: Constriction of arterioles
B: Capillary endothelial cell enlargement
C: Influx of macrophages
D: Influx of mast cells
E: Influx of polymorphs

☐ Correct Answer: *E*

Learning Response A: Incorrect. The arterioles dilate.

Learning Response B: Incorrect. The endothelial cells separate and make the basement membrane accessible to the polymorphs.

Learning Response C: Incorrect. Macrophages are in the minority in acute inflammation.

Learning Response D: Incorrect. Mast cells, unlike basophils, do not migrate to a significant extent but their degranulation mediates acute inflammatory reactions.

Learning Response E: Correct. The polymorphs are chemotactically attracted to the site of inflammation by C5a and mast cell chemotactic factors such as leukotriene B4 subset.

---

10. SUBJECT AREA: Humoral defenses
QUESTION: Lysozyme:

A: Is a cytoplasmic organelle
B: Activates complement
C: Is a proteolytic enzyme
D: Splits peptidoglycan
E: Is released by mast cells

☐ Correct Answer: *D*

Learning Response A: Incorrect. Lysozyme is a protein present in extracellular fluids and in certain granules of professional phagocytic cells.

Learning Response B: Incorrect.

Learning Response C: Incorrect.

Learning Response D: Correct. Splits the peptidoglycan of bacterial cell walls.

Learning Response E: Incorrect.

11. SUBJECT AREA: Humoral defenses
QUESTION: Which of the following is *not* an acute phase protein:

    A: Serum amyloid P component
    B: Chondroitin sulfate
    C: C-reactive protein
    D: Mannose-binding protein
    E: Fibrinogen

☐ Correct Answer: *B*

Learning Response A: Incorrect. This is an acute phase reactant whose concentration increases dramatically on infection.

Learning Response B: Correct.

Learning Response C: Incorrect. This acute phase reactant binds to certain bacterial polysaccharides and activates the first component of complement.

Learning Response D: Incorrect. This is a major acute phase protein which binds to mannose on bacteria, fixes complement, and facilitates adherence to macrophages.

Learning Response E: Incorrect. Fibrinogen shows a moderate increase in concentration on infection.

12. SUBJECT AREA: Humoral defenses
QUESTION: Interferon:

    A: Inhibits viral replication
    B: Phosphorylates a protein synthesis initiation factor
    C: Inhibits gene transcription
    D: Does all of the above (A-C)
    E: Does just two of the above (A & B)

☐ Correct Answer: *E*

Learning Response A: Incorrect. Although true, the answer is not as complete as answer E.

Learning Response B: Incorrect. Although true, not as complete a response as answer E.

Learning Response C: Incorrect. It leads to reduction in mRNA translation and the degradation of both viral and host mRNA.

Learning Response D: Incorrect.

Learning Response E: Correct.

---

13. SUBJECT AREA: Extracellular killing
QUESTION: Natural killer (NK) cells do not:

  A: Respond to interferon
  B: Contain a perforin
  C: Contain tumor necrosis factor (TNF)
  D: Kill by damaging the target cell outer membrane
  E: Contain serine proteases

☐ Correct Answer: *D*

Learning Response A: Incorrect. Their activity is stimulated by interferon.

Learning Response B: Incorrect. They contain a perforin which is released on contact with a target, inserts itself into the target cell membrane, and helps to cause lysis.

Learning Response C: Incorrect. The TNF contributes to the killer function.

Learning Response D: Correct. See learning responses B & C. The perforin insert may facilitate entry of TNF and serine proteases into the target cell.

Learning Response E: Incorrect.

---

14. SUBJECT AREA: Extracellular killing
QUESTION: Eosinophils do not:

A: Stain with basic dyes
B: Contain a major basic protein
C: Contain peroxidase
D: Give a respiratory burst on activation
E: Have C3b receptors

☐ Correct Answer: *A*

Learning Response A: Correct. They do stain with acidic dyes.

Learning Response B: Incorrect. The secreted basic protein damages protozoal membranes.

Learning Response C: Incorrect. The peroxidase contributes to the generation of reactive oxygen intermediates.

Learning Response D: Incorrect. There is a respiratory burst involving oxygen neutralization.

Learning Response E: Incorrect. The C3b receptors will bind opsonized microorganisms.

15.
SUBJECT AREA: Core revision
QUESTION: Microorganisms are kept out of the body by factors such as:

A: Skin
B: Gastric acid
C: Mucous secretion
D: All of the above
E: None of the above (A-C)

☐ Correct Answer: *D*

Learning Response A: Incorrect. Although true, answer D is more complete. Damage to skin renders the host vulnerable to infection.

Learning Response B: Incorrect. Although true, not as complete an answer as D.

Learning Response C: Incorrect. High pH is inimical to microorganisms.

Learning Response D: Correct.

Learning Response E: Incorrect.

16. SUBJECT AREA: Core revision
QUESTION: Polymorphonuclear neutrophils attack bacteria:

- A: Exclusively by oxygen-dependent mechanisms
- B: Exclusively by oxygen-independent mechanisms
- C: By phagocytosis
- D: By secreting complement
- E: By secreting interferon

☐ Correct Answer: *C*

Learning Response A: Incorrect. The production of reactive oxygen intermediates is not the only mechanism of attack.

Learning Response B: Incorrect. The oxygen-independent mechanism such as nitric oxide, defensins and so on are not the only mechanisms of attack.

Learning Response C: Correct. The ability to ingest bacteria and kill them is a major feature of these professional phagocytic cells. Loss of neutrophils renders the host very susceptible to overwhelming infection.

Learning Response D: Incorrect. Macrophages but not neutrophils secrete a number of complement components.

Learning Response E: Incorrect. Interferon is active against viruses.

17. SUBJECT AREA: Core revision
QUESTION: The complement component that is strongly chemotactic for polymorphs is:

- A: C3a
- B: C5a
- C: C3
- D: C3b
- E: C5b

☐ Correct Answer: *B*

Learning Response A: Incorrect. However, C3a is an anaphylatoxin which releases chemotactic agents such as leukotriene B_4 from mast cells.

Learning Response B: Correct. C5a is a powerful chemotactic agent and also an anaphylatoxin.

Learning Response C: Incorrect. C3 has no direct biological action but is split to give C3a and C3b when the complement system is activated by either alternative or classical pathways.

Learning Response D: Incorrect. C3b opsonizes microorganisms for adherence to phagocytic cells.

Learning Response E: Incorrect. C5b initiates formation of the membrane attack complex.

---

18. SUBJECT AREA: Core revision
QUESTION: Acute inflammation can be *initiated* by:

    A: Mast cell activation
    B: Influx of polymorphs
    C: An increase in vascular permeability
    D: C3
    E: Lysozyme

☐ Correct Answer: *A*

Learning Response A: Correct. Activation of mast cells releases chemotactic factors for polymorphs and also vasoactive mediators such as histamine.

Learning Response B: Incorrect. The influx of polymorphs represents part of the acute inflammatory response itself.

Learning Response C: Incorrect. The increase in vascular permeability is an essential feature of the acute inflammatory response itself.

Learning Response D: Incorrect. C3 has no biological activity before being cleaved.

Learning Response E: Incorrect. Lysozyme has nothing to do with acute inflammation although it may be released from polys and participate in intracellular killing within polymorphs during the phagocytic process.

---

19. SUBJECT AREA: Core revision
QUESTION: Antiviral effects are shown by:

A: C-reactive protein
B: Mannose-binding protein
C: Lysozyme
D: Interferon
E: Complement

☐ Correct Answer: *D*

Learning Response A: Incorrect. This acute phase protein binds to carbohydrate of certain bacteria and fixes C1q.

Learning Response B: Incorrect. This binds to the carbohydrate of many different microorganisms and fixes complement to facilitate phagocytosis.

Learning Response C: Incorrect. Lysozyme splits the peptidoglycan wall of susceptible bacteria.

Learning Response D: Correct. Interferon inhibits intracellular viral replication.

Learning Response E: Incorrect. However, complement can opsonize viruses for uptake by phagocytic cells.

20. SUBJECT AREA: Core revision
QUESTION: Virally infected cells can be killed directly by:

A: C5a
B: Interferon
C: NK cells
D: Eosinophils
E: C-reactive protein

☐ Correct Answer: *C*

Learning Response A: Incorrect. C5a is a mediator of the acute inflammatory reaction but does not affect virally infected cells.

Learning Response B: Incorrect. Interferon inhibits intracellular viral replication but does not kill the infected cell.

Learning Response C: Correct. NK cells bind to cells infected by some but not all viruses. There is cell to cell contact with the target and killing is by a combination of perforins, TNF, and serine proteases.

Learning Response D: Incorrect. Eosinophils are particularly potent killers of helminths.

Learning Response E: Incorrect. C-reactive protein is an acute phase reactant which has antibacterial action.

---

21. SUBJECT AREA: Complement
QUESTION: The initial complement component activated by complement-fixing antibodies is:

   A: C1q
   B: C1s
   C: C3b
   D: C5a
   E: C9

☐ Correct Answer: *A*

Learning Response A: Correct. The constant region of IgM and of most IgG antibodies binds C1q after the antibody has complexed with antigen. This eventually leads to the generation of a C4b2b convertase which splits C3.

Learning Response B: Incorrect. C1s binds only after C1q and C1r have bound.

Learning Response C: Incorrect. C3b can be generated by either the classical or alternative pathway C3 convertase and acts as an opsonin as well as being itself a part of the alternative pathway C3 convertase and of C5 convertase.

Learning Response D: Incorrect. C5a is generated by C5 convertase and acts as a powerful chemotoxin for polymorphs and an anaphylatoxin causing degranulation of mast cells.

Learning Response E: Incorrect. C9 is the final component in the complement cascade and, under the influence of C5-8, polymerizes to form part of the membrane attack complex (MAC).

---

22. SUBJECT AREA: Core revision
QUESTION: Activation of complement is a property of which antibody region:

   A: Variable
   B: Fab

C: F(ab')$_2$
D: Constant
E: Hinge

☐ Correct Answer: *D*

Learning Response A: Incorrect. The variable region is the part that binds antigen.

Learning Response B: Incorrect. The Fab region comprises one antigen-binding arm of the antibody molecule, consisting of an entire light chain and the variable region plus the first constant domain of the heavy chain.

Learning Response C: Incorrect. The F(ab')$_2$ region comprises both antigen-binding arms of the antibody molecule.

Learning Response D: Correct. The constant region does not have any role to play in binding antigen but, rather, mediates the effector functions of antibody, complement fixation, and binding to the cell surface Fc receptors on phagocytic and other cells.

Learning Response E: Incorrect. The hinge region gives the antibody molecule flexibility but is not directly involved in either antigen binding or in the effector functions of the antibody.

23. SUBJECT AREA: Complement
QUESTION: Several of the complement components are:

A: Glycolipids
B: Cell surface molecules of lymphocytes
C: Enzymes
D: Hormones
E: Antibodies

☐ Correct Answer: *C*

Learning Response A: Incorrect. The complement components are all proteins or glycoproteins.

Learning Response B: Incorrect. Although they may become deposited on the cell surface following activation, they are normally present in soluble form in blood and tissue fluids.

Learning Response C: Correct. They act in a sequential proteolytic cascade which gives tremendous amplification of the response.

Learning Response D: Incorrect. The complement components are produced by several different cell types and do not function as hormones.

Learning Response E: Incorrect. Antibodies are the specific recognition molecules which bind antigen.

---

24. SUBJECT AREA: Complement
QUESTION: The classical and alternative pathways meet at complement component:

A: C4
B: C4b
C: Factor D
D: C5
E: C3

☐ Correct Answer: *E*

Learning Response A: Incorrect. C4 is only found in the classical pathway. Note that the complement components are numbered in the order they were first identified rather than the order in which they act.

Learning Response B: Incorrect. C4b is produced by cleavage of C4 by C1qrs and forms part of the classical pathway of complement activation.

Learning Response C: Incorrect. Factor D is found in the alternative pathway and cleaves factor B in the C3bB complex to produce C3bBb, the alternative pathway C3 convertase.

Learning Response D: Incorrect. C5 is one of the later complement components which upon being split by C5 convertase forms the anaphylatoxin C5a and may go on to form the membrane attack complex containing complement components C5b, C6, C7, C8 and C9.

Learning Response E: Correct. Both pathways of complement activation produce a C3 convertase, either C4b2b (classical pathway) or C3bBb (alternative pathway), which cleaves C3 into C3a and C3b.

25. SUBJECT AREA: Core revision
QUESTION: Which cell type produces antibodies:

      A: Macrophages
      B: T lymphocytes
      C: NK cells
      D: Plasma cells
      E: Large granular lymphocytes

☐ Correct Answer: *D*

Learning Response A: Incorrect. Macrophages are phagocytic cells which are able to bind the Fc portion of antibodies but do not produce antibodies themselves.

Learning Response B: Incorrect. T lymphocytes form part of the adaptive immune response and are usually required to help in antibody production, but do not themselves produce antibody.

Learning Response C: Incorrect. NK cells are able to directly lyse target cells in the absence of antibody.

Learning Response D: Correct. B lymphocytes form part of the small lymphocyte population and have antibody on their cell surface which acts as an antigen receptor. Upon activation they differentiate into plasma cells which secrete large amounts of antibody.

Learning Response E: Incorrect. Large granular lymphocytes include NK cells which are able to directly kill certain target cells.

26. SUBJECT AREA: Core revision
QUESTION: Clonal selection occurs when a B lymphocyte encounters:

      A: Cytokines
      B: Antigen
      C: T lymphocytes
      D: Complement
      E: Chemotactic factors

☐ Correct Answer: *B*

Learning Response A: Incorrect. Cytokines are involved in clonal proliferation and maturation but not in selection.

Learning Response B: Correct. Antigen selects the few B lymphocytes, out of many millions, which have cell surface antibody which best 'fits' the antigen.

Learning Response C: Incorrect. T lymphocytes are themselves subject to clonal selection by antigen.

Learning Response D: Incorrect. Complement has several functions (e.g., chemotaxis, anaphylaxis, membrane lysis) but is not involved in clonal selection.

Learning Response E: Incorrect. Chemotactic factors attract cells, particularly phagocytes, along a concentration gradient towards, for example, the site of an infection.

---

27. SUBJECT AREA: Cellular basis of antibody production
QUESTION: A plasma cell secretes:

A: Antibody of identical specificity to that on the surface of the parent B cell
B: Antibody of two antigen specificities
C: The antigen it recognizes
D: Many different types of antibody
E: Lysozyme

☐ Correct Answer: *A*

Learning Response A: Correct. A single plasma cell secretes millions of molecules of antibody but they are all identical to the single specificity of antibody used as the antigen receptor on the B lymphocyte from which the plasma cell was derived.

Learning Response B: Incorrect. A plasma cell secretes antibody of a single specificity. Although antibodies have two antigen binding arms, they both have identical specificity.

Learning Response C: Incorrect. It secretes the antibody which the antigen recognizes.

Learning Response D: Incorrect. A plasma cell secretes antibody of a single specificity.

Learning Response E: Incorrect. Lysozyme is an antimicrobial enzyme which is produced by phagocytic cells, not plasma cells.

---

28. SUBJECT AREA: Cellular basis of antibody production
QUESTION: Specific antibodies are readily detectable in serum following primary contact with antigen:

   A: After 10 minutes
   B: Within 1 hour
   C: By 5-7 days
   D: After 3-5 weeks
   E: Until a second contact with antigen

☐ Correct Answer: *C*

Learning Response A: Incorrect. Following antigen selection the B lymphocyte requires time to proliferate in order to expand up the clone of cells, some of which then differentiate into antibody-secreting plasma cells.

Learning Response B: Incorrect. Following antigen selection, the B lymphocyte requires time to proliferate in order to expand up the clone of cells, some of which then differentiate into antibody-secreting plasma cells.

Learning Response C: Correct. Five days or more are required for B-cell proliferation, maturation, and the secretion of a large enough amount of antibody for it to be readily detected systemically.

Learning Response D: Incorrect. By 3-5 weeks the level of specific antibody is declining.

Learning Response E: Incorrect. Although a greater amount of antibody is produced following the second contact with antigen, appreciable amounts are produced following primary contact.

---

29. SUBJECT AREA: Core revision
QUESTION: The secondary, but not the primary, immune response is based on:

   A: Memory
   B: The bonus effect of multivalency
   C: Complement activation

D: Mast cell degranulation
  E: Clonal selection

☐ Correct Answer: A

Learning Response A: Correct. The clonal proliferation that occurs during a primary immune response produces both effector lymphocytes and memory cells. These memory cells constitute an expanded population of specific lymphocytes which form the basis of the secondary immune response.

Learning Response B: Incorrect. This concept refers to the fact that antibodies are at least bivalent with respect to antigen binding, and antigenic epitopes are often multivalent. These multivalent interactions greatly increase the functional affinity (avidity) of binding.

Learning Response C: Incorrect. Complement activation is not directly responsible for secondary immune responses, although C3 in immune complexes aids localization of antigen in germinal centers where secondary responses occur.

Learning Response D: Incorrect. Mast cell degranulation is involved in acute inflammatory type I hypersensitivity reactions.

Learning Response E: Incorrect. Clonal selection refers to the binding by antigen of lymphocytes with a complementary receptor; this occurs in both primary and secondary immune responses.

---

30. SUBJECT AREA: Acquired immunity has antigen specificity
QUESTION: Antibodies against an individual's own body components are called:

  A: Isotypes
  B: Autoantigens
  C: Autoantibodies
  D: Primary
  E: Interferons

☐ Correct Answer: C

Learning Response A: Incorrect. Isotypes refer to the class of antibody (e.g., IgM, IgG).

Learning Response B: Incorrect. Refers to antigens which comprise the body's own constituents, not antibodies against these antigens.

Learning Response C: Correct. Antibodies which bind to any normal body constituent are called autoantibodies.

Learning Response D: Incorrect. This term describes the type of immune response obtained after an initial encounter with antigen.

Learning Response E: Incorrect. These are soluble mediators with antiviral and immunomodulatory activities.

---

31. SUBJECT AREA: Vaccination depends on acquired memory
QUESTION: Edward Jenner vaccinated against smallpox using:

        A: Killed smallpox virus
        B: A recombinant protein derived from smallpox
        C: An unrelated virus
        D: Toxoid
        E: Cowpox

☐ Correct Answer: *E*

Learning Response A: Incorrect. Note, however, that killed virus is used in some present day vaccines against other infectious agents, e.g., whooping cough and polio.

Learning Response B: Incorrect. The term recombinant protein is used to refer to a molecule produced using recombinant DNA technology, not available 200 years ago!

Learning Response C: Incorrect. An unrelated virus would be unlikely to share antigens with smallpox and therefore would be of no use as a vaccine for this disease.

Learning Response D: Incorrect. Toxoids are chemically modified non-pathogenic bacterial toxins which can be used as vaccines against the harmful effects of the corresponding bacteria by eliciting antibodies which neutralize the toxin.

Learning Response E: Correct. The smooth unblemished skin of milkmaids gave Jenner the idea of using cowpox. The cowpox virus is non-virulent in man but shares antigens with the related smallpox virus and is therefore able to elicit protection against subsequent infection with smallpox.

32. SUBJECT AREA: Vaccination depends on acquired memory
QUESTION: Protective antibodies against infectious agents are often:

        A: Autoantibodies
        B: Neutralizing
        C: Toxoids
        D: NK cells
        E: Non-specific

☐ Correct Answer: *B*

Learning Response A: Incorrect. These are antibodies against 'self' molecules.

Learning Response B: Correct. They protect by neutralizing a function of the pathogen such as the harmful part of a toxin or a viral coat protein which binds to a cell-surface viral receptor on the host cells.

Learning Response C: Incorrect. Toxoids are chemically-modified non-pathogenic bacterial toxins which can be used as vaccines against the harmful effects of the corresponding bacteria by eliciting antibodies which neutralize the toxin.

Learning Response D: Incorrect. Natural killer is a type of large granular lymphocyte which is able to kill certain target cells such as tumor cells and some virally-infected cells.

Learning Response E: Incorrect. All antibodies, irrespective of the type of antigen they recognize, are defined by and have their protective action through their specificity for that antigen.

33. SUBJECT AREA: Acquired memory
QUESTION: Adoptive transfer of acquired immune responsiveness involves the transfer of:

        A: Antibody
        B: Complement
        C: Phagocytes
        D: Lymphocytes
        E: Serum

☐ Correct Answer: *D*

Learning Response A: Incorrect. Experimental situations in which antibody, or antibody-containing serum, is transferred from one experimental animal to another is referred to as *passive* transfer of immunity.

Learning Response B: Incorrect. Experimentally, complement components may be transferred to, e.g., complement-deficient strains of mice, in order to help confirm the role of that component. However, this does not transfer acquired immune responsiveness.

Learning Response C: Incorrect. Adoptive transfer can be used to transfer immunological memory to a naive recipient but phagocytic cells are not the cell type responsible for the enhanced immune response which occurs on the second encounter with specific antigen.

Learning Response D: Correct. Adoptive transfer experiments helped establish that immunological memory, one of the hallmarks of the adaptive immune response, is a property of the small lymphocyte.

Learning Response E: Incorrect. Experimental situations in which antibody-containing serum is transfered from one experimental animal to another is referred to as *passive* transfer.

---

34. SUBJECT AREA: Cellular basis of antibody production
QUESTION: Paul Ehrlich's theory of antibody production was called:

- *A:* Side-chain
- *B:* Template
- *C:* Clonal selection
- *D:* Opsonization
- *E:* B cell

☐ Correct Answer: *A*

Learning Response A: Correct. He proposed that each cell would make a large variety of surface receptors ('side-chains') which bound foreign antigens by complementarity of shape in a 'lock-and-key' fit; side-chains which bound antigen would increase in number. Even though he proposed this as long ago as 1894 he was almost right. What he did not predict was that each cell had 'side-chains' (i.e., antibody) of only a single specificity.

Learning Response B: Incorrect. This hypothesis was proposed later by other scientists to explain the vast range of antibody specificities that the immune system can generate. The idea was that the antigen acted as a template around which the antibody folded. Although this turned out to be wrong, it was a reasonable idea at a time when dogma stated one gene–one protein.

Learning Response C: Incorrect. The clonal selection theory was proposed by Sir MacFarlane Burnett who conceived that each antibody-producing cell (B cell) could produce, and had on its surface, antibodies of a single specificity. The clone of B cells bearing the antibody that fitted the antigen best were selected to proliferate and further differentiate.

Learning Response D: Incorrect. Opsonization refers to the ability of antibody and/or complement components to enhance phagocytosis of the organism or molecule they coat.

Learning Response E: Incorrect. We now know that B cells make antibody, but in Ehrlich's time little was known about the cells which produced the antibody.

35.
SUBJECT AREA: Core revision
QUESTION: Secondary antibody reponses are better because:

A: They have a broader specificity
B: They make mainly IgM antibody
C: Complement-fixing antibodies are made
D: They do not require T-cell help
E: They are stronger and faster

☐ Correct Answer: *E*

Learning Response A: Incorrect. Both primary and secondary immune responses are specific for the antigen which elicits the response. A secondary immune response only occurs if the same antigen is encountered as that which produced the primary immune response.

Learning Response B: Incorrect. IgM is the major antibody class made during the initial stages of an immune response, but in a secondary immune response, most of the antibody made is IgG or IgA.

Learning Response C: Incorrect. Both IgM (found mainly in the primary immune response) and IgG (found mainly in the secondary immune response) antibodies are efficient at complement fixation.

Learning Response D: Incorrect. Secondary immune responses require T cells which provide help, mainly in the form of cytokines, in order for the B cells to make antibody. In fact, antigens which provoke antibody responses in the absence of T cells ('T-independent antigens') are unable to elicit a secondary type of immune response but rather stimulate a primary type of immune response no matter how many times they are encountered.

Learning Response E: Correct. Upon the second encounter with the same antigen, the response occurs much quicker, the amount of antibody made is much greater, and the response lasts longer. This forms the basis for vaccination, using a harmless form of the infective agent for the initial injection.

36.

SUBJECT AREA: Acquired memory

QUESTION: The main reason an experimental animal treated with x-rays can act as a living test tube for lymphocyte transfer experiments is because:

- *A:* It is microbiologically sterile
- *B:* Complement components will be inactivated
- *C:* The host lymphocytes are destroyed or unable to divide
- *D:* Only non-dividing cells are affected
- *E:* The requirement for T-cell help is overcome

☐ Correct Answer: C

Learning Response A: Incorrect. Although x-irradiation can be used to kill microorganisms, this is not the reason it is used in lymphocyte transfer experiments, which utilize a comparatively low level of irradiation.

Learning Response B: Incorrect. The doses of irradiation used are too low to cause any substantial damage to complement.

Learning Response C: Correct. Lymphocytes are highly sensitive to radiation and if the host's lymphocytes are destroyed or unable to divide following treatment with x-rays, then any immune response observed following lymphocyte transfer will be of donor, not recipient, origin.

Learning Response D: Incorrect. It is dividing cells which are affected by irradiation.

Learning Response E: Incorrect. X-irradiation does not overcome a requirement for T-cell help and therefore for an antibody response to a T-cell dependent antigen to occur in the recipient, both T and B lymphocytes must be transferred.

37. SUBJECT AREA: Acquired immunity has antigen specificity
QUESTION: Immunological unreponsiveness to self antigens is called:

       A: Tolerance
       B: Tolerogen
       C: Memory
       D: Acquired immunity
       E: ADCC

☐ Correct Answer: *A*

Learning Response A: Correct. Tolerance is a specific immunological non-responsiveness. Although tolerance can be induced to any antigen, the mechanism is thought to have evolved as a means of preventing the maturation of self-reactive lymphocytes.

Learning Response B: Incorrect. A tolerogen is an antigen capable of inducing a state of tolerance. Most antigens are capable of acting as tolerogens. Whether the outcome of an initial encounter with antigen results in an immune response or tolerance depends on several criteria including the amount of antigen (very high or very low doses are often tolerogenic), route of administration, and the form in which the antigen is given (e.g., monomeric or polymeric).

Learning Response C: Incorrect. Memory is the phenomenon whereby the immune system is able to recall a previous encounter with a given antigen and thus mount a secondary immune response. The term 'recall antigen' is sometimes used to denote common antigens capable of eliciting strong secondary immune responses (e.g., tetanus toxoid, candida).

Learning Response D: Incorrect. Acquired immunity is used to differentiate the adaptive immune system from the innate immune system, and refers to the fact that the immune system acquires a large range of specificities based on antigen receptor gene rearrangement followed by exposure of lymphocytes to a broad range of environmental antigens.

Learning Response E: Incorrect. ADCC refers to a phenomenon called antibody-dependent cell-mediated cytotoxicity. This is a mechanism for killing target cells coated with antibody, but instead of a complement-mediated or phagocytic attack, Fc receptor–bearing cells such as monocytes and NK cells recognize the antibody-coated target cells and then kill the target by delivering a 'lethal hit.'

38. Subject area: Core revision
Question: Protection against microorganisms inside cells is provided by:

- A: T cells
- B: IgG
- C: IgM
- D: Complement
- E: The membrane attack complex

☐ Correct Answer: A

Learning Response A: Correct. T lymphocytes are specialized for recognizing peptides derived from intracellular infectious agents which are exhibited on the surface of an infected cell together with MHC class I and II molecules.

Learning Response B: Incorrect. Appreciable amounts of antibody are not normally able to enter cells, although Fc receptor-mediated endocytosis of immune complexes containing IgG does occur.

Learning Response C: Incorrect. IgM is a large molecule (970 kDa) and is unable to enter cells.

Learning Response D: Incorrect. Complement is a powerful weapon in the immune system armamentarium and plays a role in protection against extracellular infection. It does not have access to intracellular infective agents.

Learning Response E: Incorrect. However, cytotoxic T lymphocytes (CTL) which do provide protection against intracellular viral infections do so by inserting a channel-forming molecule called perforin into the cell membrane in a way very similar to that seen with the membrane attack complex (MAC), and complement component C9 and perforin show significant sequence homology.

39. Subject area: Cell-mediated immunity protects against intracellular organisms
Question: Intracellular parasites within macrophages are killed more readily in the presence of:

- A: Antibody
- B: Kinins
- C: Properdin
- D: γ Interferon
- E: Anaphylatoxin

☐ Correct Answer: *D*

Learning Response A: Incorrect. Generally speaking, antibodies do not readily enter cells and therefore intracellular parasites are inaccessible to antibodies. Fc receptor-mediated internalization of antibody does occur, but even then the antibody is thought to be confined within endocytotic vesicles and would not be able to attack intracellular parasites.

Learning Response B: Incorrect. Kinins are vasoactive peptides that are produced following tissue injury.

Learning Response C: Incorrect. Properdin binds to and stabilizes C3bBb in the alternative pathway of complement activation.

Learning Response D: Correct. γ Interferon activates microbicidal mechanisms within the macrophage, thereby leading to the death of intracellular parasites.

Learning Response E: Incorrect. The anaphylatoxins are molecules such as the complement components C3a and C5a which trigger mast cell degranulation.

40. SUBJECT AREA: Immunopathology
QUESTION: Thyrotoxicosis is:

- *A:* An allergic reaction to a drug
- *B:* A phenomenon seen following transplant rejection
- *C:* An immune response to tetanus toxoid
- *D:* A form of T-cell negative selection in the thymus
- *E:* An autoimmune disease

☐ Correct Answer: *E*

Learning Response A: Incorrect. This is a tissue-damaging hypersensitivity reaction to an exogenous antigen.

Learning Response B: Incorrect. Graft rejection is an undesirable consequence of the immune system, but is a completely artificial situation which has only come about with the advent of advanced surgical techniques.

Learning Response C: Incorrect. A toxoid is an inactivated form of a bacterial toxin.

Learning Response D: Incorrect. The thymus is a primary lymphoid organ and a major site of T-cell development.

Learning Response E: Correct. Thyrotoxicosis is an autoimmune disease in which, rather than being protective against foreign organisms ('non-self'), the immune system attacks the body's own components ('self'), in this case producing stimulatory autoantibodies against the TSH receptor in the thyroid gland.

41. SUBJECT AREA: Ig structure
QUESTION: The basic Ig unit is composed of:

      A: 2 identical heavy and 2 identical light chains
      B: 2 identical heavy and 2 different light chains
      C: 2 different heavy and 2 identical light chains
      D: 2 different heavy and 2 different light chains
      E: Non-covalently bound peptide chains

☐ Correct Answer: *A*

Learning Response A: Correct.

Learning Response B: Incorrect. Once a given light (or heavy) chain has been successfully rearranged, the other light (or heavy) chain gene complexes remain unrearranged. Thus only one light and one heavy chain is expressed, a phenomenon known as allelic exclusion.

Learning Response C: Incorrect. See learning response B.

Learning Response D: Incorrect. See learning response B.

Learning Response E: Incorrect. The heavy and light chains are mostly linked by interchain disulfide bonds although when these are reduced, heavy and light chains only separate when exposed to extreme conditions such as high pH.

42. SUBJECT AREA: Ig structure
QUESTION: A Fab fragment:

      A: Is produced by pepsin treatment
      B: Is produced by separation of heavy and light chains
      C: Binds antigen
      D: Lacks light chains
      E: Has no interchain disulfide bonds

☐ Correct Answer: C

Learning Response A: Incorrect. Pepsin treatment produces the divalent F(ab')$_2$ through splitting C-terminal to the disulfide bond linking the two heavy chains.

Learning Response B: Incorrect. The Fab fragment produced by papain splitting the hinge region N-terminal to the inter-heavy chain disulfide bond, includes the light chain and only a portion of the heavy chain.

Learning Response C: Correct. Fab = fragment antigen binding.

Learning Response D: Incorrect. The Fab consists of a light chain and the V_H and C_{H1} domains of the heavy chain.

Learning Response E: Incorrect. The disulfide bonds linking the light and part of the heavy chain are present.

43. SUBJECT AREA: Ig structure
QUESTION: The complementarity determining regions:

- A: Are restricted to light chains
- B: Are in the constant part of the Ig molecule
- C: Bind to Fc receptors
- D: Are concerned in antigen recognition
- E: Occur at the C-terminal end of the Ig peptide chains

☐ Correct Answer: D

Learning Response A: Incorrect. The three complementarity determining regions in the variable part of the light chain contribute to antigen binding.

Learning Response B: Incorrect. They are in the variable regions.

Learning Response C: Incorrect. Being in the variable regions, they cannot bind to Fc receptors.

Learning Response D: Correct. Three CDRs in the heavy and 3 in the light chain may all be concerned in forming the antigen recognition structure.

Learning Response E: Incorrect. They occur at the N-terminal region.

44. SUBJECT AREA: Ig genes
QUESTION: Which of the following gene clusters do not contribute to antigen binding:

    A: V_L
    B: C_L
    C: V_H
    D: D
    E: J

☐ Correct Answer: *B*

Learning Response A: Incorrect. V_L genes are involved in antigen binding.

Learning Response B: Correct. The constant region genes encoding the constant region of the light chain do not bear antigen binding CDRs.

Learning Response C: Incorrect.

Learning Response D: Incorrect. The D segments do contribute through recombination with V and J segments to form antigen binding variable regions.

Learning Response E: Incorrect. The J segments contribute through recombination with V and D segments to form antigen binding variable regions.

---

45. SUBJECT AREA: Ig genes
QUESTION: Translocation of V, D and J Ig gene segments:

    A: Only occurs in mature B cells
    B: Only occurs in light chains
    C: Involves heptamer-spacer-heptamer flanking sequences
    D: Does not occur until the mRNA stage
    E: Is effected by recombinase enzymes

☐ Correct Answer: *E*

Learning Response A: Incorrect. A translocation only occurs in developing immature B cells.

Learning Response B: Incorrect. The light chain gene complex does not contain D minisegments.

Learning Response C: Incorrect. It involves heptamer-spacer-nonamer flanking sequences.

Learning Response D: Incorrect. It involves translocation of DNA gene segments.

Learning Response E: Correct.

46.
SUBJECT AREA: Ig structural variants
QUESTION: Allelic forms of Ig are referred to as:

  A: Idiotypes
  B: Isotypes
  C: Allotypes
  D: Subclasses
  E: Subgroups

☐ Correct Answer: C

Learning Response A: Incorrect. Idiotypes are the collection of epitopes on the variable region of an immunoglobulin which are recognized by a collection of antibodies directed against them (the so-called anti-idiotypic serum).

Learning Response B: Incorrect. Isotypes such as IgG, IgA, etc., are present in all normal individuals of a given species.

Learning Response C: Correct. These genetically alternative forms of immunoglobulin are not present in all individuals.

Learning Response D: Incorrect. Subclasses such as IgG1, IgG2 and so on, are present in all individuals. They are isotypes.

Learning Response E: Incorrect. Subgroups represent framework families of variable region genes which are present in all normal individuals.

47.
SUBJECT AREA: Ig domains
QUESTION: With reference to the variable Ig domains, which of these answers is false:

  A: It mediates the secondary consequences of antigen recognition
  B: It has anti-parallel β-pleated sheet structures

C: It uses β-turn loops to bind antigen
D: It has an extra long β-turn relative to constant region domains
E: It has a typical Ig fold with an intra-chain disulfide bond.

☐ Correct Answer: A

Learning Response A: Correct. This is a devious question because the correct implies that the statement is false. The variable domains recognize antigen and secondary consequences of this are mediated by the Fc region composed of the C-terminal segments of the heavy chains.

Learning Response B: Incorrect. The statement is true.

Learning Response C: Incorrect. The statement is true.

Learning Response D: Incorrect. The statement is true.

Learning Response E: Incorrect. The statement is true.

48. SUBJECT AREA: Ig domains
QUESTION: The C-terminal domain of IgG heavy chain (Cγ3) is termed:

A: F(ab')$_2$
B: Fc
C: pFc'
D: Fv
E: Fd

☐ Correct Answer: C

Learning Response A: Incorrect. F(ab')$_2$ refers to the divalent antigen binding fragment obtained after pepsin treatment.

Learning Response B: Incorrect. The Fc non-antigen binding region is made up of the Cγ2 and Cγ3 C-terminal domains of the heavy chain.

Learning Response C: Correct. This results after pepsin treatment of IgG which destroys the Cγ2 domain.

Learning Response D: Incorrect. This represents the two variable region domains of heavy and light chains. It has a single binding site for antigen.

Learning Response E: Incorrect. The Fd represents the V and Cγ1 domains of the heavy chain.

49. SUBJECT AREA: Ig classes
QUESTION: Which of the following statements does *not* apply to IgG:

- *A:* Appears early in the immune response
- *B:* Neutralizes bacterial toxins
- *C:* Can fix complement
- *D:* Crosses the human placenta
- *E:* Opsonizes bacteria

☐ Correct Answer: *A*

Learning Response A: Correct. Another tricky question where the false statement is a correct response. IgM is the class which appears early.

Learning Response B: Incorrect.

Learning Response C: Incorrect.

Learning Response D: Incorrect.

Learning Response E: Incorrect.

50. SUBJECT AREA: Ig classes
QUESTION: The low affinity FcγRII IgG receptor:

- *A:* Is present on NK cells
- *B:* Binds monomeric IgE
- *C:* Binds monomeric IgG
- *D:* Binds aggregated IgG
- *E:* Is not present on macrophages

☐ Correct Answer: *D*

Learning Response A: Incorrect. The NK receptor is the low affinity FcγRIII-A.

Learning Response B: Incorrect. The receptor does not cross-react with IgE.

Learning Response C: Incorrect. Because of its low affinity, there is no appreciable binding of the monomer.

Learning Response D: Correct. Although low affinity, aggregated IgG binds in a multivalent fashion and gains by the bonus effect of this multivalent binding.

Learning Response E: Incorrect.

---

51. SUBJECT AREA: Ig classes
QUESTION: IgA in seromucous secretions:

- *A:* Has no J-chain
- *B:* Has no secretory piece
- *C:* Is dimeric
- *D:* Cannot bind to polymorphs
- *E:* Activates the classical complement pathway

☐ Correct Answer: *C*

Learning Response A: Incorrect.

Learning Response B: Incorrect. The secretory piece is that part of the poly-Ig receptor bound to the dimeric IgA which remains after cleavage following transport across the glandular epithelial cell.

Learning Response C: Correct. The molecule dimerizes within the plasma cell so that the 4 valencies are identical and the multivalency assists binding to polymeric bacterial and other antigens.

Learning Response D: Incorrect. Polymorphs have Fcα receptors.

Learning Response E: Incorrect.

---

52. SUBJECT AREA: Ig classes
QUESTION: IgM:

- *A:* Is usually of high affinity
- *B:* Is tetrameric
- *C:* Normally adopts a 'crab'-like configuration
- *D:* Is a weak bacterial agglutinator
- *E:* Is the main class of the 'natural antibodies'

☐ Correct Answer: *E*

Learning Response A: Incorrect. IgM is usually of low affinity but because of its many valencies, i.e., combining sites for antigen, it is of a high avidity for a polymeric antigen.

Learning Response B: Incorrect. It is pentameric.

Learning Response C: Incorrect. Normally has a star-like configuration but adopts the crab-like structure when bound to a polymeric antigen.

Learning Response D: Incorrect. It is a strong bacterial agglutinator because of its multivalency.

Learning Response E: Correct. The natural antibodies, which include many anti-bacterial antibodies, arise largely without external antigenic stimulation. In the mouse they are made by the $CD5^+$ B1 subset.

53.
SUBJECT AREA: Ig classes
QUESTION: IgD:

- *A:* Is pentameric
- *B:* Is resistant to proteolytic degradation
- *C:* Is present mainly as a surface receptor on B cells
- *D:* Is present with unusual frequency in myelomas
- *E:* Is abundant in milk

☐ Correct Answer: C

Learning Response A: Incorrect. It is monomeric.

Learning Response B: Incorrect. It is highly susceptible to proteolysis.

Learning Response C: Correct. It has the same specificity as the surface IgM receptor.

Learning Response D: Incorrect. It very rarely occurs as a myeloma protein.

Learning Response E: Incorrect. IgA is abundant in milk.

54.
SUBJECT AREA: Ig classes
QUESTION: IgE:

    A: Is abundant in saliva
    B: Binds strongly to mast cells
    C: Cannot bind to macrophages
    D: Activates the complement cascade
    E: Has an insignificant role in worm infestations

☐ Correct Answer: *B*

Learning Response A: Incorrect. It is at a very low concentration in the body fluids. IgA is predominant in saliva.

Learning Response B: Correct. The Fcε receptor on mast cells binds IgE very strongly and cross-linking by antigen leads to mast cell activation and initiation of an inflammatory reaction.

Learning Response C: Incorrect. There are low affinity Fcε receptors on macrophages.

Learning Response D: Incorrect.

Learning Response E: Incorrect. IgE antibodies play an important role in defense against worm infection.

55.
SUBJECT AREA: Ig classes
QUESTION: Which IgG subclass fixes complement strongly but lacks the Ga rheumatoid factor site and fails to bind staphylococcal protein A:

    A: IgG1
    B: IgG2
    C: IgG3
    D: IgG4
    E: None of the above

☐ Correct Answer: *C*

Learning Response A: Incorrect.

Learning Response B: Incorrect.

Learning Response C: Correct.

Learning Response D: Incorrect.

Learning Response E: Incorrect.

---

56. SUBJECT AREA: Core revision
QUESTION: The number of different peptide chains in a basic immunoglobulin molecule is:

    A: 1
    B: 2
    C: 3
    D: 4
    E: 5

☐ Correct Answer: *B*

Learning Response A: Incorrect.

Learning Response B: Correct. There are 2 identical heavy chains and 2 identical light chains.

Learning Response C: Incorrect.

Learning Response D: Incorrect. There are a total of 4 peptide chains in the basic Ig molecule but they are only of 2 different types.

Learning Response E: Incorrect.

---

57. SUBJECT AREA: Core revision
QUESTION: Cleavage of IgG by papain produces:

    A: Divalent antigen binding fragments
    B: Light chains
    C: Heavy chains
    D: F(ab')$_2$
    E: Fab

☐ Correct Answer: *E*

Learning Response A: Incorrect. Monovalent antigen binding fragments are produced.

Learning Response B: Incorrect. Light chains can be separated from heavy chains by reduction of the interchain disulfide bonds.

Learning Response C: Incorrect. See learning response B.

Learning Response D: Incorrect. The divalent antigen binding fragment, F(ab')$_2$ is produced by pepsin and there is loss of the Fc region.

Learning Response E: Correct. Papain splits the hinge sequences above the inter-heavy chain disulfide bond and produces a monovalent antigen binding fragment consisting of light chain and part of the heavy chain containing the V_H and C_{H1} domains.

58.
SUBJECT AREA: Core revision
QUESTION: A given myeloma protein:

- A: Has a homogeneous amino acid structure
- B: Has a variable peptide segment
- C: Has a constant heavy chain but both κ and λ light chains
- D: Is produced by different plasma cell clones
- E: Does not behave as an antibody

☐ Correct Answer: *A*

Learning Response A: Correct. A given myeloma protein is the product of a single clone of cancer cells all producing an immunoglobulin with identical peptide structure.

Learning Response B: Incorrect. See learning response A.

Learning Response C: Incorrect. Constant heavy chain is associated with either κ or λ light chains but never both.

Learning Response D: Incorrect. The myeloma protein is a product of a single plasma cell clone which has proliferated without regard for the host.

Learning Response E: Incorrect. It is an immunoglobulin and as such can function as an antibody although very often the antigen has not been identified.

59. SUBJECT AREA: Core revision
QUESTION: What is the approximate size of the gene cluster giving rise to the D region:

A: 1000
B: 100
C: 50
D: 4
E: 1

☐ Correct Answer: *D*

Learning Response A: Incorrect.

Learning Response B: Incorrect.

Learning Response C: Incorrect.

Learning Response D: Correct.

Learning Response E: Incorrect.

---

60. SUBJECT AREA: Core revision
QUESTION: Recombinase enzymes effect the translocation of:

A: V to J
B: V to D
C: D to J
D: All of the above
E: V to λ

☐ Correct Answer: *D*

Learning Response A: Incorrect. True but not as complete an answer as D. Random translocation of V, D and J mini-segments greatly increases the number of variable region structures and hence specificities for antigen.

Learning Response B: Incorrect. True but not as complete as D. See learning response A.

Learning Response C: Incorrect. See learning response A.

Learning Response D: Correct.

Learning Response E: Incorrect. The joining of variable to constant regions takes place by splicing at the mRNA level.

---

61. SUBJECT AREA: Core revision
QUESTION: A given Ig isotype is:

A: A heavy chain variant encoded by allelic genes
B: A light chain constant region encoded by allelic genes
C: Present in all normal individuals
D: A collection of hypervariable region epitopes recognized by an anti-idiotype
E: Monoclonal

☐ Correct Answer: *C*

Learning Response A: Incorrect. These polymorphic forms are termed allotypes and being genetically controlled, are not necessarily present in each individual.

Learning Response B: Incorrect. See learning response A.

Learning Response C: Correct. Isotypes like immunoglobulin classes or subclasses are all expressed in normal individuals.

Learning Response D: Incorrect. This is the definition of an idiotype.

Learning Response E: Incorrect. Any given immunoglobulin constant region isotype is connected to a whole variety of different variable regions and therefore to that extent is extensively polyclonal.

---

62. SUBJECT AREA: Core revision
QUESTION: The Fab region of an Ig is responsible for:

A: Complement fixation
B: Binding to antigen
C: Binding to Fc receptors
D: Binding to macrophages
E: The ability of Ig to cross the human placenta

☐ Correct Answer: *B*

Learning Response A: Incorrect. Complement fixation is effected by the Fc region which is separated from the Fab fragments when the Ig molecule is split by papain at the hinge region.

Learning Response B: Correct. Fab equals fragment antigen binding and is monovalent because it has a single site for antigen binding.

Learning Response C: The Fab is distinct from the Fc and therefore cannot bind to the Fc receptors.

Learning Response D: Incorrect. The binding of macrophages occurs through the Fc region.

Learning Response E: Incorrect. Crossing the placenta is mediated by binding of immunoglobulin to Fcγ receptors.

---

63. SUBJECT AREA: Core revision
QUESTION: The main Ig in the seromucous secretions defending the external body surfaces is:

A: IgG
B: IgD
C: IgE
D: IgM
E: IgA

☐ Correct Answer: *E*

Learning Response A: Incorrect. IgG is the main immunoglobulin in the body fluids.

Learning Response B: Incorrect. IgD is present almost entirely as a B lymphocyte surface receptor.

Learning Response C: Incorrect. IgE coating mast cells is a second line of defense of external body surfaces when they have been penetrated by an infectious agent.

Learning Response D: Incorrect. IgM is largely intravascular.

Learning Response E: Correct. Secreted IgA which is dimeric and has secretory piece is the main defensive Ig in the seromucous secretions.

---

64. SUBJECT AREA: The B-cell surface receptor for antigen
QUESTION: The first immunoglobulin heavy chain class to be expressed on the surface of a newly produced B cell is:

A: IgA
B: IgD
C: IgE
D: IgG
E: IgM

☐ Correct Answer: *E*

Learning Response A: Incorrect. IgA is found later on in the immune response following 'class switching' and is particularly associated with mucosal immunity.

Learning Response B: Incorrect. Although IgD is found on the membrane early on in the development of B cells, it is not the first immunoglobulin to be expressed.

Learning Response C: Incorrect. IgE occurs later on in the immune response following 'class switching' and is particularly associated with mucosal immunity.

Learning Response D: Incorrect. IgG is found later on in the immune response following 'class switching' and is the major immunoglobulin class in serum and in the tissues.

Learning Response E: Correct. IgM is the first immunoglobulin class to be expressed on the surface of the developing B cells, shortly followed by IgD. Early mature B cells co-express IgM and IgD antibodies of identical antigen specificity.

---

65. SUBJECT AREA: The B-cell surface receptor for antigen
QUESTION: A B cell is able to make cell-surface and secreted versions of antibody using:

A: Different gene pools
B: Alternative splicing
C: Different heavy chain class but the same light chain
D: Different light chain class but the same heavy chain
E: F(ab')$_2$ fragments

☐ Correct Answer: *B*

Learning Response A: Incorrect. The gene pools used for the cell-surface and secreted antibodies are identical.

Learning Response B: Correct. Differential (alternative) splicing of a primary RNA transcript can produce antibody either with or without exons encoding a hydrophobic transmembrane sequence which leads to retention of antibody in the cell surface membrane.

Learning Response C: Incorrect. In a given B cell, heavy chains of different classes (e.g., IgM and IgD) can combine with the same light chain, although not in a single antibody molecule. However, the heavy chain class does not determine whether the antibody will be cell-surface associated or secreted.

Learning Response D: Incorrect. In a given B cell the antibody heavy chains are always associated with the same light chains. Note that recent evidence suggests that during early B-cell development if the antibody produced reacts against 'self,' the B cell may be able to express a different light chain and be given the opportunity of avoiding tolerance induction mechanisms if the new heavy–light combination no longer reacts with self, a phenomenon referred to as receptor editing.

Learning Response E: Incorrect. F(ab')$_2$ fragments lack the transmembrane sequence (and all but one of the heavy chain constant region domains) of the antibody but are produced artificially in the laboratory by digestion with the proteolytic enzyme pepsin and do not occur naturally in vivo.

66. SUBJECT AREA: The B-cell surface receptor for antigen
QUESTION: The cytoplasmic region of surface IgM consists of:

        A: A single H chain constant region domain
        B: A light chain
        C: 110 amino acids
        D: 3 amino acids
        E: Carbohydrate

☐ Correct Answer: *D*

Learning Response A: Incorrect. IgM possesses four heavy chain constant region domains, but these all lie extracellularly.

Learning Response B: Incorrect. The light chains are disulfide-bonded to the transmembrane heavy chains but are not themselves directly held in the membrane and therefore do not possess any cytoplasmic regions.

Learning Response C: Incorrect. This is the size of an immunoglobulin domain.

Learning Response D: Correct. This is too short to directly transmit a signal into the cell following antigen binding, a function carried out by accessory molecules.

Learning Response E: Incorrect. IgM is glycosylated but only on the extracellular part of the molecule.

---

67. SUBJECT AREA: Core revision
QUESTION: The molecules mediating signal transduction following antigen binding to cell surface immunoglobulin on a virgin B cell are called:

A: Ig Fc
B: IgM-α and Ig-β
C: MHC
D: CD4
E: CD8

☐ Correct Answer: *B*

Learning Response A: Incorrect. The Fc part of a cell surface antibody molecule contains a short cytoplasmic tail but this is not responsible for signal transduction.

Learning Response B: Correct. IgM-α and Ig-β possess C-terminal cytoplasmic regions which become phosphorylated upon cross-linking of membrane immunoglobulin, leading to a rapid mobilization of intracellular calcium.

Learning Response C: Incorrect. MHC molecules are specialized for the presentation of antigenic peptides to the T-cell receptor.

Learning Response D: Incorrect. CD4 molecules are found on a subpopulation of T cells, but not on B cells, and they recognize MHC class II molecules.

Learning Response E: Incorrect. CD8 molecules are found on a subpopulation of T cells, but not on B cells, and they recognize MHC class I molecules.

68. SUBJECT AREA: Core revision
QUESTION: The T-cell receptor for antigen is:

      A: Derived from the immunoglobulin gene pool by alternative splicing
      B: A tetramer
      C: A homodimer
      D: A heterodimer
      E: A single chain molecule

☐ Correct Answer: D

Learning Response A: Incorrect. The immunoglobulin and T-cell receptor molecules are encoded by entirely separate gene pools.

Learning Response B: Incorrect. Unlike immunoglobulin molecules, which are tetramers made up of two identical heavy chains and two identical light chains.

Learning Response C: Incorrect. T-cell receptor molecules, on mature T cells at least, are dimers but the chains are not identical.

Learning Response D: Correct. There are two versions of the T-cell receptor, both of which are heterodimers consisting of an α chain and a β chain, or a γ chain and a δ chain.

Learning Response E: Incorrect. Although a number of T-cell surface molecules are single chain structures, e.g., Thy-1 and CD4, the T-cell receptor is not.

69. SUBJECT AREA: Core revision
QUESTION: Each chain of the T-cell receptor consists of:

      A: An Ig heavy chain
      B: Two Ig-type domains
      C: A fibronectin-type domain
      D: Glycolipid molecules
      E: Four Ig-type domains

☐ Correct Answer: B

Learning Response A: Incorrect. The antigen receptor of T lymphocytes (the T-cell receptor) and of B lymphocytes (antibody) do not have any chains in common.

Learning Response B: Correct. Immunoglobulin-type domains are found in a large number of cell surface and soluble molecules, some of which fulfill roles in the immune system (e.g., immunoglobulins, T-cell receptors, MHC, CD4, CD8) but many of which are found elsewhere such as in the nervous system.

Learning Response C: Incorrect. Many molecules, particularly those involved in adhesion, have fibronectin-type domains, but the T-cell receptor does not.

Learning Response D: Incorrect. T-cell receptor molecules are glycoproteins.

Learning Response E: Incorrect. However, the heavy chains of IgG, IgA and IgD do have four Ig superfamily domains (one variable and three constant), whilst IgM and IgE have five (one variable and four constant).

---

70. SUBJECT AREA: The T-cell surface receptor for antigen
QUESTION: The T-cell receptor genes were originally identified using:

        A: A monoclonal anti-idiotype
        B: The polymerase chain reaction
        C: A liver DNA gene library
        D: In situ hybridization
        E: Subtractive hybridization

☐ Correct Answer: *E*

Learning Response A: Incorrect. Such a reagent was used to identify clonally-restricted receptors on the surface of T lymphocytes, but not to identify the genes encoding these molecules.

Learning Response B: Incorrect. In fact, the PCR technique was first described in 1985, one year after the first reports of the cloning of T-cell receptor genes.

Learning Response C: Incorrect. Although a liver DNA gene library would contain all the T-cell receptor genes in a given individual, these would be in the germ line (unrearranged) configuration and would not be expressed as mRNA. The original discovery of the T-cell receptor genes relied on identifying genes that were rearranged in T cells.

Learning Response D: Incorrect. In situ hybridization can be used to identify genes expressed in individual cells, but was not utilized in the discovery of the T-cell receptor genes.

Learning Response E: Correct. Given that the vast majority of the mRNA in B-cells encodes molecules also expressed in T cells, subtractive hybridization was used as a step in the initial identification of the T-cell receptor. This technique removed from a T-cell polysomal mRNA preparation all of the mRNA molecules also present in B-cells, leaving a T-cell specific series of clones, some of which hybridized to DNA which was rearranged only in mature T cells.

71. SUBJECT AREA: The T-cell surface receptor for antigen
QUESTION: The percentage of human peripheral blood T-cells bearing a γδ T-cell receptor is:

  A: 30-80%
  B: 0.5-15%
  C: 100%
  D: 0%
  E: Only present during mycobacterial infections

☐ Correct Answer: *B*

Learning Response A: Incorrect. However, this figure would be correct for the percentage of peripheral blood γδ T cells in ruminants.

Learning Response B: Correct. Although they constitute a minority of the peripheral blood T cells in man, γδ T cells are more heavily represented in intestinal epithelium and in skin.

Learning Response C: Incorrect. Human peripheral blood T cells comprise both αβ and γδ subsets.

Learning Response D: Incorrect. γδ T cells are present in human peripheral blood.

Learning Response E: Incorrect. Although γδ T cells seem to be strongly biased towards recognition of mycobacterial antigen, they are normally present irrespective of mycobacterial infection.

72. SUBJECT AREA: The T-cell surface receptor for antigen
QUESTION: A chromosome on which T-cell receptor α chain gene rearrangement has occurred lacks which of the following gene segments:

A: Joining (J)
B: Diversity (D)
C: Variable (V)
D: Constant (C)
E: TCR β chain

☐ Correct Answer: *B*

Learning Response A: Incorrect. The Jα gene segment to which a Vα gene segment has rearranged, together with all the Jα gene segments 3' of that to which the rearrangement occurred, will be present.

Learning Response B: Correct. The T-cell receptor α chain genes do not possess D gene segments, although the δ chain genes do. However, because the δ chain locus is found entirely within the α chain locus and is located between the Vα and the Jα gene segments, any α chain gene rearrangements lead to the loss of the δ chain gene segments, including all of the Dδ segments.

Learning Response C: Incorrect. The Vα gene segment which has rearranged, together with all the remaining 5' Jα gene segments, will be present.

Learning Response D: Incorrect. The Cδ gene which lies within the T-cell receptor α chain gene locus will be lost but the single Cα gene will still be present.

Learning Response E: Incorrect. The T-cell receptor α chain and β chain genes are encoded on separate chromosomes.

73. SUBJECT AREA: Core revision
QUESTION: The T-cell receptor antigen recognition signal is transduced by:

A: The TCR α chain
B: The TCR β chain
C: CD1
D: CD2
E: CD3

☐ Correct Answer: *E*

Learning Response A: Incorrect. Like immunoglobulin, the T-cell receptor does not itself transduce a signal to the inside of the lymphocyte.

Learning Response B: Incorrect. Like immunoglobulin, the T-cell receptor does not itself transduce a signal to the inside of the lymphocyte.

Learning Response C: Incorrect. CD1 is a molecule which is involved in antigen presentation to γδ T cells.

Learning Response D: Incorrect. CD2 forms a signalling unit on the surface of T cells, but does not transduce the signal for the T-cell receptor.

Learning Response E: Correct. CD3 is a molecule composed of five polypeptide chains (CD3-γ, -δ, and -ε plus ζ-ζ, η-η or ζ-η), which transduces the antigen recognition signal received by the T-cell receptor heterodimer to the inside of the cell.

74. SUBJECT AREA: The generation of diversity for antigen recognition
QUESTION: Using only random VDJ recombination, from 100 V, 4 D and 6 J gene segments, the number of possible variable regions of an antigen receptor molecule would be:

A: 100
B: 110
C: 2,400
D: 10^6
E: 10^9

☐ Correct Answer: *C*

Learning Response A: Incorrect. The variable region of the protein is encoded by three separate gene segments, V, D and J, not solely by one of the V (variable) gene segments.

Learning Response B: Incorrect. Random combination gives more than the arithmetical summation of the individual gene segments. If this were not the case there would be little point in employing the complex VDJ recombination strategy used by the antigen receptor genes.

Learning Response C: Correct. 100 × 4 × 6 = 2,400. The use of geometric random recombination enables a much larger number of different molecules to be produced than would otherwise be possible.

Learning Response D: Incorrect. This is much greater than would be produced solely by random recombination of the specified number of genes, but purely by combining 2,400 heavy chains with 350 different possible κ light chains would produce this number of different immunoglobulin molecules. The addition of λ light chains would make this number even greater.

Learning Response E: Incorrect. This is an estimated potential diversity of heavy:light chain combinations based not solely on random VDJ (for heavy chain) and VJ (for light chain) but also on additional mechanisms that are used to create diversity.

---

75. SUBJECT AREA: The generation of diversity for antigen recognition
QUESTION: N-region insertion is associated with the expression of:

- *A:* Terminal deoxynucleotidyl transferase
- *B:* Somatic hypermutation
- *C:* The proteasome
- *D:* Lysozyme
- *E:* Heat shock proteins

☐ Correct Answer: *A*

Learning Response A: Correct. This enzyme mediates the insertion of nucleotides at the N-region of the D and J gene segments.

Learning Response B: Incorrect. This is also a process for increasing antibody diversity but is different from N-region insertion.

Learning Response C: Incorrect. This is an enzyme complex involved in the processing of cytosolic protein antigens into short peptides for subsequent presentation by MHC molecules to T cells.

Learning Response D: Incorrect. This is an enzyme with anti-microbial activity due to its ability to digest bacterial cell wall peptidoglycan.

Learning Response E: Incorrect. Evolutionarily highly conserved molecules involved in chaperone functions, these are not involved in N-region insertion.

76. SUBJECT AREA: Core revision
QUESTION: Somatic hypermutation is:

- A: Found in both Ig and T-cell receptor genes
- B: Restricted to the constant region
- C: Restricted to the hypervariable regions
- D: Found only in Ig heavy chains
- E: Found only in Ig variable regions

☐ Correct Answer: *E*

Learning Response A: Incorrect. Somatic hypermutation has not been observed in T-cell receptor genes, possibly because the requirement to recognize self-MHC could lead to high affinity self-reactivity if somatic hypermutation were to take place.

Learning Response B: Incorrect. Somatic hypermutation is not found in the constant region genes, suggesting a very precise targetting of the hypermutation process.

Learning Response C: Incorrect. Somatic hypermutation is common in, but not restricted to, the hypervariable (complementarity-determining) regions.

Learning Response D: Incorrect. Somatic hypermutation takes place in the genes encoding both the heavy and the light chains of immunoglobulin.

Learning Response E: Correct. Somatic hypermutation is restricted to the variable region of immunoglobulin and is found in both the hypervariable and the framework regions.

77. SUBJECT AREA: The major histocompatibility complex (MHC)
QUESTION: The MHC class II region genes in the mouse are located:

- A: On a different chromosome to the class I region genes
- B: On a different arm, but on the same chromosome, as the class I region genes
- C: On chromosome 6
- D: Adjacent to a class I gene
- E: In the HLA locus

☐ Correct Answer: *D*

Learning Response A: Incorrect. All the MHC genes are located on the same chromosome.

Learning Response B: Incorrect. All the MHC genes lie adjacent to each other.

Learning Response C: Incorrect. The MHC genes in man are on chromosome 6 but in the mouse are on chromosome 17.

Learning Response D: Correct. The MHC class II genes in mouse, H-2A and H-2E, are located in between a class I gene, H-2K, and the MHC class III genes.

Learning Response E: Incorrect. The MHC in mouse is termed H-2; HLA is the human MHC.

---

78. SUBJECT AREA: The major histocompatibility complex (MHC)
QUESTION: The MHC class I heavy chain consists of:

- A: β_2-microglobulin
- B: Three Ig-type domains
- C: A truncated MHC class II heavy chain
- D: Three globular domains
- E: Two globular domains

☐ Correct Answer: *D*

Learning Response A: Incorrect. β_2-microglobulin constitutes the MHC class I light chain (11 kDa) which is noncovalently linked to the transmembrane heavy (α) chain.

Learning Response B: Incorrect. There is only one immunoglobulin-type domain in the MHC class I heavy chain.

Learning Response C: Incorrect. The class I and class II molecules are encoded by different genes.

Learning Response D: Correct. They consist of one membrane-proximal immunoglobulin-type domain and two membrane-distal domains which form a grooved structure comprising two extended α-helices lying on top of a β-pleated sheet floor.

Learning Response E: Incorrect. Each chain of the MHC class II molecule comprises an immunoglobulin-type domain and a membrane distal domain which, together with the membrane-distal domain on the other chain, forms a grooved structure comprising two extended α-helices lying on top of a β-pleated sheet floor.

79. SUBJECT AREA: The major histocompatibility complex (MHC)
QUESTION: The MHC class II β chain has a molecular weight of:

   A: 28 kDa
   B: 34 kDa
   C: 43-44 kDa
   D: 11 kDa
   E: 25 kDa

☐ Correct Answer: A

Learning Response A: Correct. Like the α chain, the β chain is a transmembrane glycoprotein with two extracellular globular domains.

Learning Response B: Incorrect. This is the size of the MHC class II α chain.

Learning Response C: Incorrect. The MHC class I α chain, weighing in at 43-44 kDa, is the largest of the chains of the classical MHC molecules.

Learning Response D: Incorrect. This is the molecular weight of β_2-microglobulin, a single immunoglobulin-type domain molecule encoded outside the MHC and which, lacking a transmembrane region, associates noncovalently with the MHC class I α chain.

Learning Response E: Incorrect. 25 kDa is the molecular weight of an immunoglobulin light chain.

80. SUBJECT AREA: The major histocompatibility complex (MHC)
QUESTION: MHC class III genes encode:

   A: Complement component C3
   B: Tumor necrosis factor
   C: IL-2
   D: β_2-microglobulin
   E: HLA-DQ

☐ Correct Answer: B

Learning Response A: Incorrect. Complement components C2, C4 and factor B are encoded within this region.

Learning Response B: Correct. Both TNFα and TNFβ are encoded within the MHC class III region.

Learning Response C: Incorrect. IL-2 is not encoded within any part of the MHC.

Learning Response D: Incorrect. β_2-microglobulin forms part of the structure of the MHC class I molecule, but is encoded outside of the MHC.

Learning Response E: Incorrect. HLA-DQ is one of the MHC class II molecules in man.

---

81. SUBJECT AREA: The major histocompatibility complex (MHC)
QUESTION: Extensive allelic polymorphism is found in MHC:

    A: DQ α
    B: DR α
    C: β_2-microglobulin
    D: Class I α_3 domain
    E: Class II β_2 domain

☐ Correct Answer: *A*

Learning Response A: Correct. Class I HLA-A and -B molecules are highly polymorphic, so are the class II molecule DQ α, DQ β and DR β chains. The DP β chain is also polymorphic but less so than the others mentioned.

Learning Response B: Incorrect. DRα is not polymorphic.

Learning Response C: Incorrect. β_2-microglobulin is not polymorphic.

Learning Response D: Incorrect. The α_1 and α_2 domains of MHC class I molecules are highly polymorphic and form the peptide-binding cleft of the molecule.

Learning Response E: Incorrect. The β_1 domain of MHC class II molecules is polymorphic and, together with the polymorphic α_1 domain of the α chain, forms the peptide-binding cleft of the molecule.

82. SUBJECT AREA: Core revision
QUESTION: MHC class II molecules are found on:

  A: Virtually all cells in the body
  B: B cells, antigen-presenting cells and macrophages
  C: Only γ-interferon activated cells
  D: Virtually all *nucleated* cells in the body
  E: Only on virally-infected cells

☐ Correct Answer: *B*

Learning Response A: Incorrect. Expression of MHC class II molecules is normally restricted to certain cell types. However they can be induced in most cell types by IFNγ.

Learning Response B: Correct. These cells are able to present processed endogenous antigen to CD4$^+$ T cells.

Learning Response C: Incorrect. γ-Interferon increases the level of MHC class I expression and induces normally absent MHC class II expression on capillary endothelium and on many epithelial cells.

Learning Response D: Incorrect. MHC class I molecules are found on virtually all nucleated cells in the body. They are expressed abundantly on lymphoid cells, less so on liver, lung and kidney, and sparsely on brain and skeletal muscle.

Learning Response E: Incorrect. MHC class I molecules on virally-infected cells will present virus-derived peptides to CD8$^+$ T cells.

83. SUBJECT AREA: The major histocompatibility complex (MHC)
QUESTION: Expression of MHC genes is:

  A: Codominant
  B: Dominant for maternal genes
  C: Dominant for paternal genes
  D: Dependent on thymic selection
  E: Dependent on the antigenic exposure of the individual

☐ Correct Answer: *A*

Learning Response A: Correct. The MHC molecules encoded by both parental genes are expressed.

Learning Response B: Incorrect. The MHC molecules encoded by both parental genes are expressed.

Learning Response C: Incorrect. The MHC molecules encoded by both parental genes are expressed.

Learning Response D: Incorrect. Thymic selection is for T cells expressing T-cell receptors which can recognize foreign peptides presented by self MHC molecules.

Learning Response E: Incorrect. The expression of MHC genes is not directly regulated by the antigenic exposure of the individual, although cytokines released by T cells responding to foreign antigen may cause an *upregulation* of MHC gene expression.

84.
SUBJECT AREA: Antigens
QUESTION: A hapten is:

- *A:* An epitope
- *B:* A paratope
- *C:* A small chemical grouping which reacts with preformed antibodies
- *D:* A carrier
- *E:* An immunogen

☐ Correct Answer: *C*

Learning Response A: Incorrect. An epitope is that region of an antigen that is in contact with a combining site of a single antibody.

Learning Response B: Incorrect. A paratope is that part of the antibody surface which is in contact with the antigen.

Learning Response C: Correct. The chemical grouping reacts with preformed antibodies including that on the specific B-cell surface but cannot induce an antibody response.

Learning Response D: Incorrect. A carrier is a protein moiety bearing T-cell epitopes which can act to provide T-cell help for a B-cell antibody response to determinants on the protein carrier or an attached chemical grouping (hapten).

Learning Response E: Incorrect. A hapten cannot stimulate an immune response even though it can react with preformed antibodies. To induce antibody formation it needs to be linked to a carrier and it would then be termed an immunogen, i.e., a molecule capable of generating an immune response. The term is sometimes restricted to those molecules which can generate not just an immune response but actually a protective response where the antigen is part of an infectious agent.

85. SUBJECT AREA: Antigens
QUESTION: A discontinuous antigen epitope is:

- *A:* An antigenic determinant
- *B:* Usually concave
- *C:* Defined by its protein structure
- *D:* Produced by a continuous linear peptide sequence
- *E:* Produced by non-adjacent amino acid residues

☐ Correct Answer: *E*

Learning Response A: Incorrect. An antigenic determinant is usually applied to a cluster of epitopes recognized by a polyclonal antiserum.

Learning Response B: Incorrect. Concave regions of the antigen surface bind water strongly and are usually very poorly immunogenic. Epitopes are usually present on the protruding parts of the antigen surface.

Learning Response C: Incorrect. Although the epitope is constructed from the peptide chain (S), the *definition* of an epitope is entirely determined by the nature of the antibody with which it combines.

Learning Response D: Incorrect. The discontinuous epitope is produced by non-adjacent amino acid residues brought together by the folding of peptide chains. Part of the epitope might have a contribution from two or three adjacent amino acid residues.

Learning Response E: Correct. Residues which may be far apart on the linear sequence of a protein may be brought close together in space by the protein folding. Denaturation of the protein will tend to result in a loss of binding power for antibody.

86. SUBJECT AREA: Antigen-antibody interaction
QUESTION: Binding of antigen to antibody:

>   A: Is usually unaffected by molecular rigidity
>   B: Is unaffected by the presence or absence of water molecules
>   C: Involves covalent bonding
>   D: Is optimized by spatial complementarity
>   E: Is usually unaffected by pH

☐ Correct Answer: *D*

Learning Response A: Incorrect. Antigen and antibody very rarely match as complementary structures exactly and flexibility allows residues to come together to give strong binding energy.

Learning Response B: Incorrect. The exclusion of water molecules is essential for the development of a hydrophobic bond between antigen and antibody. The high dielectric constant of water greatly reduces the Coulombic attraction of opposite charges on antigen and antibody. If water molecules intervene between two charges, Van der Waals forces only become great when antigen and antibody are in close electron cloud apposition and this is unlikely if water molecules intervene. Where positive or negative charges are not balanced by an opposite charge on the ligand, water molecules lower the free energy of the system and may be found interspersed between antigen and antibody.

Learning Response C: Incorrect. The antigen-antibody bonds are entirely reversible which would not be the case if there were covalent bonding such as occurs in disulphide bonds for example.

Learning Response D: Correct. Spatial complementarity is vital for strong binding of antigen to antibody so that the otherwise non-specific intermolecular forces, which depend reciprocally on distance apart, can become really strong.

Learning Response E: Incorrect. A change in pH either adds or subtracts hydrogen ions from antigen and antibody, depending on the direction of the pH change, and this will cause a conformational alteration in the protein folding and also make both proteins bare similar charges. This leads to a lowering of affinity.

87. SUBJECT AREA: Antigen-antibody interaction
QUESTION: The intermolecular forces which contribute to the interaction include:

A: Electrostatic
B: Van der Waals
C: Hydrophobic
D: All of the above (A-C)
E: Only 2 of the above (A&C)

☐ Correct Answer: D

Learning Response A: Incorrect. Electrostatic interactions between opposite charges do contribute but this answer is not as complete as that of D.

Learning Response B: Incorrect. Van der Waals' forces representing interaction between electron clouds on antigen and antibody do contribute to binding and are very strong at small intermolecular distances. However this answer is not as complete as that of D.

Learning Response C: Incorrect. Hydrophobic bonding between groups of antigen and antibody which do not hydrogen bond with water, contributes to antigen-antibody binding. However this answer is not as complete as that of D.

Learning Response D: Correct.

Learning Response E: Incorrect.

88. SUBJECT AREA: Antigen-antibody interaction
QUESTION: Which of the following statements is *incorrect*? Affinity is:

A: A measure of the strength of the binding of antigen to antibody
B: The association constant of the Ag/Ab equilibrium
C: Avidity
D: Related to the free energy change of the Ag/Ab interaction
E: Related to specificity

☐ Correct Answer: C

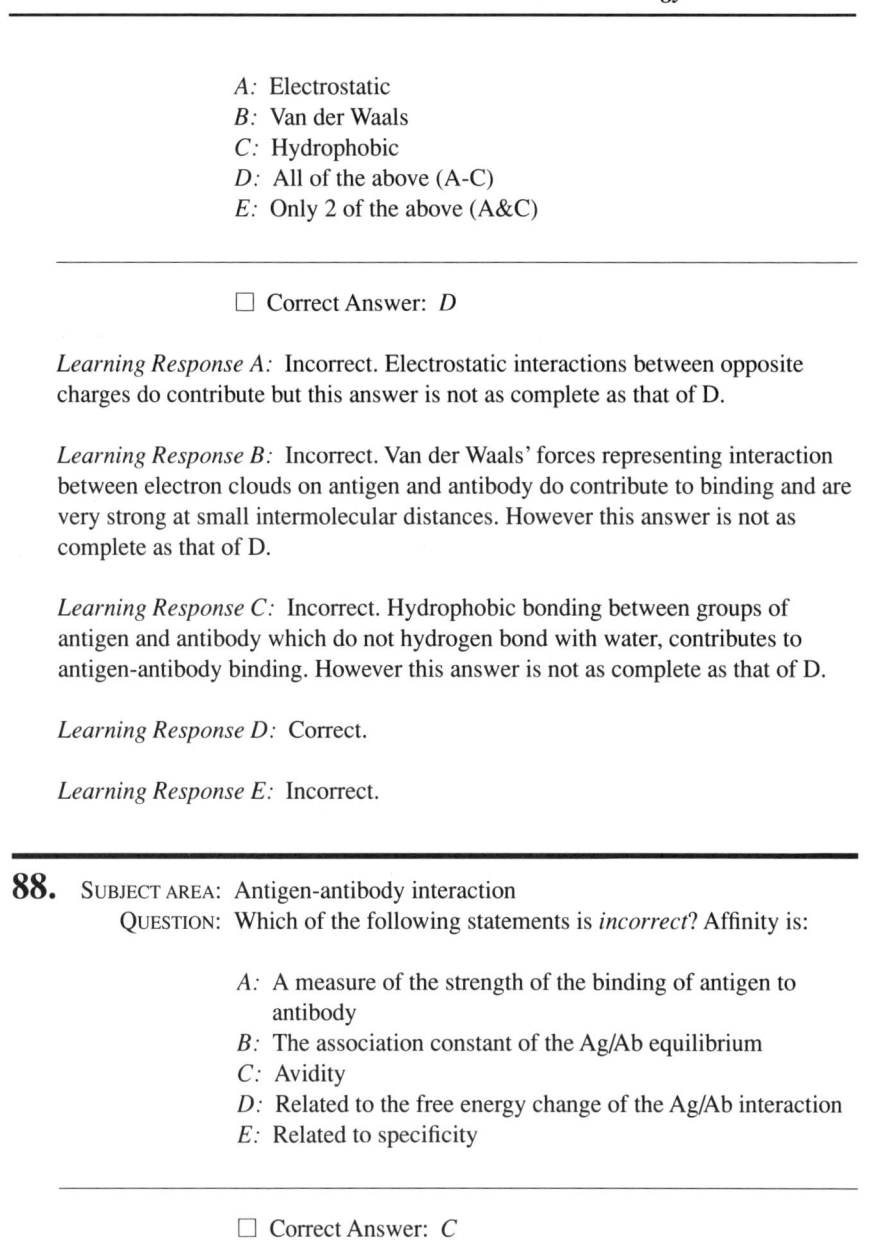

Learning Response A: Incorrect. This statement is true. Affinity measures the strength of binding of epitope to paratope.

Learning Response B: Incorrect. The statement is true. Affinity is the equilibrium constant of the formation of paratope/epitope complex. The reciprocal is the dissociation constant. Affinities can be expressed as either.

Learning Response C: Correct. This statement is untrue because avidity refers to the functional "affinity" of the interaction between a complex antigen and its antiserum containing several different specific antibodies. Where antigens are held together by two or more bonds or an antibody binds to an antigen with two or more bonds, the binding strength (i.e., the avidity) is much greater than the component affinities due to the bonus effect of multivalency.

Learning Response D: Incorrect. This statement is true. The relationship is $\delta G = -RTl_{nk}$, where δG is the free energy change, R the gas constant, T absolute temperature and k the affinity.

Learning Response E: Incorrect. This is a true statement. The ability of antibody to discriminate between two antigens is related to the relative affinity for each of the antigens.

89.
SUBJECT AREA: T-cell recognition
QUESTION: The antigen moiety on an antigen-presenting cell recognized by the T-cell receptor is:

- A: Native protein antigen plus major histocompatibility complex (MHC) molecule
- B: Processed (peptide) antigen plus MHC
- C: Processed peptide antigen
- D: Native antigen
- E: MHC alone

☐ Correct Answer: *B*

Learning Response A: Incorrect. The native protein antigen does not combine with the MHC. The T cell wants to recognize processed not native antigen.

Learning Response B: Correct. The peptide in the MHC groove is derived from intracellular proteins, either endogenous or exogenously derived.

Learning Response C: Incorrect. The peptide antigen by itself without the MHC does not signal a cellular origin.

Learning Response D: Incorrect. Native antigen is not an indicator of an intracellular infective agent and is normally recognized extracellularly by antibody.

Learning Response E: Incorrect. The MHC is present all the time and that signal alone within the body is only a signal of normality.

90. SUBJECT AREA: T-cell recognition
QUESTION: The processing of cytosolic protein involves:

    A: Transport into late endosomes
    B: Proteasome-mediated cleavage
    C: Displacement of invariant chain
    D: Displacement of β_2-microglobulin
    E: Binding to the MHC class II groove

☐ Correct Answer: *B*

Learning Response A: Incorrect. Exogenously derived proteins are processed within endocytic vesicles and become acidic late endosomes before fusion with MHC class II derived from the ER.

Learning Response B: Correct. The cytosolic proteins are cleaved to small peptides in the proteasome complex before they are transported by the TAP-1/2 molecules into the endoplasmic reticulum.

Learning Response C: Incorrect. Fusion with late endosomes leads to displacement of the invariant chain from its union with the nascent MHC class II molecules. Thereafter, appropriate peptides within the fused vacuoles combine with the MHC class II groove.

Learning Response D: Incorrect. The processed cytosolic proteins give rise to peptides which reinforce the stability of the β_2-microglobulin/class I heavy chain complex.

Learning Response E: Incorrect. The cytosolic protein after processing binds to the MHC class I groove within the endoplasmic reticulum before transport to the surface.

91. SUBJECT AREA: T-cell recognition
QUESTION: The processed peptide binding to the MHC class I groove:

    A: Is usually more than 11 amino acids long
    B: Hangs over the ends of the groove
    C: Usually binds to the groove through 2 anchor residues

D: Is mainly recognized by the CDR1 of the T-cell receptor chains
E: Is derived from exogenous protein taken in by endocytosis

☐ Correct Answer: *C*

Learning Response A: Incorrect. The processed peptide fitting to the class I groove is usually 8-11 amino acids long.

Learning Response B: Incorrect. The peptide sits within the MHC class I groove and if it is slightly long, it kinks up in the middle.

Learning Response C: Correct. Each polymorphic MHC class I molecule has two major pockets associated with the groove which bind strongly to side chains on the processed peptide.

Learning Response D: Incorrect. The CDR1 is mainly concerned in recognition of the MHC helix and groove. Peptide is recognized more by the CDR3 regions.

Learning Response E: Incorrect. The exogenous proteins are degraded and finish up in the MHC class II groove. Processed cytosolic proteins are bound finally to the MHC class I groove.

92. SUBJECT AREA: T-cell recognition
QUESTION: Superantigens:

A: Do not cause pathology
B: Are mitogenic for B cells
C: Bind to MHC class I
D: Bind to all members of a given Vβ T-cell receptor family
E: Have to be processed before recognition by the T cell

☐ Correct Answer: *D*

Learning Response A: Incorrect. Superantigens of the streptococcal exotoxin type cause diphtheria, vomiting and fever.

Learning Response B: Incorrect. They are very powerfully mitogenic for T cells bearing certain Vβ families but do not react with B cells to cause proliferation.

Learning Response C: Incorrect. Superantigens bind to MHC class II non-polymorphic sites.

Learning Response D: Correct. They recognize the common structures in a given Vβ T-cell receptor family and bind to all of them, cross-linking the T cell to the MHC class II on an antigen-presenting cell. This is a powerful stimulus.

Learning Response E: Incorrect. They combine with the T-cell Vβ receptor in their native state and do not require processing.

93. SUBJECT AREA: Difference in B- and T-cell recognition
QUESTION: T cells recognize MHC plus processed peptide:

        A: To eliminate extracellular organisms
        B: To avoid self-reactivity
        C: To scavenge unwanted metabolic products
        D: To directly kill viruses
        E: To recognize an intracellular infection

☐ Correct Answer: *E*

Learning Response A: Incorrect. Extracellular organisms are eliminated by antibody largely working in collaboration with complement. Antibody therefore has to see the native conformation on the live organism.

Learning Response B: Incorrect. Self-reactivity is only avoided if the processed peptide is present together with the MHC in appreciable concentrations in contact with the developing T cells within the thymus gland.

Learning Response C: Incorrect. Unwanted metabolic products are either eliminated through secretion or are bound by a variety of antibodies including natural antibodies in the circulation.

Learning Response D: Incorrect. The T cell does not recognize a virus directly. It sees peptide derived from intracellular virus associated with MHC and can kill the virally infected cell before the virus has had time to replicate significantly.

Learning Response E: Correct. T cells deal directly cell to cell with an infected cell, either through cytotoxicity or by release of appropriate cytokines such as the macrophage activating interferon-γ. In order to recognize an intracellular infection, it uses the code, MHC = cell, processed peptide = infectious agent within the cell.

94. SUBJECT AREA: Core revision
QUESTION: An epitope:

- A: Is the area on an antigen which contacts antibody
- B: Is the area on an antibody which contacts antigen
- C: Is an antigenic determinant
- D: Is usually composed of a linear sequence of amino acids
- E: Is usually associated with a concave region of the antigen

☐ Correct Answer: A

Learning Response A: Correct. It refers to a single antibody not a polyclonal antiserum.

Learning Response B: Incorrect. This is called a paratope. It contacts the epitope on the antigen.

Learning Response C: Incorrect. An antigenic determinant usually refers to a cluster of epitopes recognized by a polyclonal antiserum.

Learning Response D: Incorrect. Most antibodies directed to a protein antigen react with a discontinuous determinant in which the residues which contact antibody are present on different segments of the peptide chain brought close together in space by the protein folding.

Learning Response E: Incorrect. Concave regions contain water which is difficult to displace and consequently these regions are poorly immunogenic unlike the convex regions.

95. SUBJECT AREA: Core revision
QUESTION: The binding strength of antigen to antibody:

- A: Is irreversible
- B: Depends on covalent interactions
- C: Depends essentially on hydrophobic bonds
- D: Depends on spatial complementarity
- E: Is measured by specificity

☐ Correct Answer: D

Learning Response A: Incorrect.

Learning Response B: Incorrect. That is why antigen antibody bonds are usually reversible.

Learning Response C: Incorrect. Although hydrophobic bonds often constitute a major fraction of the binding energy, Coulombic hydrogen bonding and Van der Waal's forces all play a part.

Learning Response D: Correct. The spatial complementarity allows antigen and antibody to approach close together in space, allowing the non-specific molecular forces to achieve relatively high values.

Learning Response E: Incorrect. The binding force is measured by affinity. Specificity measures the relative affinities for the two different antigens being compared.

---

96. SUBJECT AREA: Core revision
QUESTION: T-cell receptors recognize:

      A: Native antigen
      B: Free linear antigenic peptide
      C: MHC β_2-microglobulin
      D: Linear antigen peptide in the MHC groove
      E: Carbohydrate antigens associated with the MHC

☐ Correct Answer: *D*

Learning Response A: Incorrect. Antibodies recognize native antigen.

Learning Response B: Incorrect. Free antigenic peptide not associated with MHC is not recognized by T-cell receptor.

Learning Response C: Incorrect. β_2-microglobulin is associated with the MHC class I heavy chain and the T-cell receptor recognizes polymorphic variants around the peptide binding groove.

Learning Response D: Correct. The peptide together with MHC is a code for intracellular infection.

Learning Response E: Incorrect. Carbohydrate antigens do not get processed to associate with the MHC.

97.
SUBJECT AREA: Core revision
QUESTION: Peptides produced by processing of cytosolic proteins largely:

- A: Are generated in late endosomal vacuoles
- B: Enter the endoplasmic reticulum by diffusion
- C: Are presented at the cell surface with MHC class II to CD4 T-helpers
- D: Are presented at the cell surface with MHC class II to CD8 cytotoxic T cells
- E: Are presented at the cell surface with MHC class I to CD8 cytotoxic T cells

☐ Correct Answer: *E*

Learning Response A: Incorrect. External proteins taken in by endocytosis are processed in endosomal vacuoles which form part of the MHC class II pathway.

Learning Response B: Incorrect. The peptides are actively transported to the endoplasmic reticulum.

Learning Response C: Incorrect. This refers to external proteins processed in late endosomal vacuoles.

Learning Response D: Incorrect. MHC class II plus peptide is not recognized by CD8 cytotoxic T cells.

Learning Response E: Correct. The CD8 molecule contacts the non-polymorphic parts of the MHC class I.

98.
SUBJECT AREA: Core revision
QUESTION: Antigenic peptides in the MHC class I groove:

- A: Are usually 12-25 residues in length
- B: Are usually 9-11 residues in length
- C: Extend beyond the groove
- D: Have 3 or more invariant anchor residues
- E: Do not vary at non-anchor residues

☐ Correct Answer: *B*

Learning Response A: Incorrect. This is the length of the residues usually associated with MHC class II grooves.

Learning Response B: Correct. The peptide fits within the groove and if it is slightly too long, kinks upwards in the middle.

Learning Response C: Incorrect. This is true of class II–associated peptides.

Learning Response D: Incorrect. The peptide usually has 2 residues which anchor it to the MHC groove.

Learning Response E: Incorrect. Variation at the non-anchor residues offers specificity for the T-cell receptor recognition.

99.
SUBJECT AREA: Core revision
QUESTION: *Staphylococcus aureus* superantigens:

    A: Do not cause pathology
    B: Are recognized by T cells in processed form
    C: Are potent T-cell mitogens
    D: Stimulate T cells independently of Vβ family
    E: Stimulate T cells independently of the presence of MHC class II accessory cells

☐ Correct Answer: *C*

Learning Response A: Incorrect. They cause food poisoning, vomiting and diarrhea.

Learning Response B: Incorrect. The superantigens are not processed but cross-link molecules onto cells in the native form.

Learning Response C: Correct. They are amongst the most potent T-cell mitogens known.

Learning Response D: Incorrect. The superantigens recognize a particular T-cell receptor Vβ family and stimulate members of that family.

Learning Response E: Incorrect. The cross-linking of T-cell receptor to the MHC class II on the accessory cell is essential for stimulation.

100. SUBJECT AREA: Core revision
QUESTION: T cells must directly recognize:

      A: Infected cells
      B: Live whole microorganisms
      C: Dead whole microorganisms
      D: Native epitopes on extracellular microorganisms
      E: Native epitopes on intracellular microorganisms

☐ Correct Answer: *A*

Learning Response A: Correct. T cells recognize MHC plus processed peptide which act as a dual code: MHC codes for cell and processed peptide is an indicator of an intracellular protein. In this way the T cell recognizes an intracellular as distinct from an extracellular infective agent.

Learning Response B: Incorrect. Since T cells must recognize infected cells, they only recognize the processed proteins as indicators of the intracellular infection.

Learning Response C: Incorrect. No point. Once dead, the microorganism should be phagocytosed and disposed of.

Learning Response D: Incorrect. Extracellular microorganisms in their native state are recognized by antibody.

Learning Response E: Incorrect. T cells recognize intracellular infection by virtue of the linear peptide derived from the microorganism lying within the MHC groove. The native protein would not fit within the MHC groove but a special mechanism processes the intracellular microorganism proteins and transports the resulting peptides to the MHC on the surface.

---

101. SUBJECT AREA: Estimation of antibody
QUESTION: Antibody titer refers to the:

      A: Absolute amount of specific antibody
      B: Affinity of specific antibody
      C: Avidity of specific antibody
      D: Concentration of total antibody
      E: Highest dilution of antibody still able to give a positive result in a test system

☐ Correct Answer: *E*

Learning Response A: Incorrect. The titer of an antiserum is not determined solely by the quantity of antibody.

Learning Response B: Incorrect. The titer of an antiserum is not determined solely by the affinity of the antibodies.

Learning Response C: Incorrect. Avidity is the functional affinity obtained when multivalency of the reactants is taken into account, but the titer of an antiserum is not determined solely by the avidity of antibodies.

Learning Response D: Incorrect. The titer of an antiserum is not determined solely by the concentration of specific antibody.

Learning Response E: Correct. The titer is determined by both the abundance and the affinity of the antigen-specifc antibodies in an antiserum and by the sensitivity of the read-out system.

---

102. SUBJECT AREA: Estimation of antibody
QUESTION: In extreme antigen excess, immune complexes have the composition:

A: Ag_1Ab_4
B: Ag_4Ab_3
C: Ag_2Ab_1
D: Ag_3Ab_2
E: Ag_2Ab_7

☐ Correct Answer: *C*

Learning Response A: Incorrect. This type of complex would be formed in antibody excess.

Learning Response B: Incorrect. This type of complex would be formed in less severe antigen excess.

Learning Response C: Correct. This is due to the bivalent nature of the antibody molecule which will be saturated in antigen excess.

Learning Response D: Incorrect. This type of complex would be formed in less severe antigen excess.

Learning Response E: Incorrect. This type of complex would be formed in antibody excess.

---

103. SUBJECT AREA: Core revision
QUESTION: Which of the following is not used for the precipitation of immune complexes:

   A: Nephelometry
   B: Polyethylene glycol
   C: Ammonium sulfate
   D: Antibody to immunoglobulin
   E: Staphylococci

☐ Correct Answer: *A*

Learning Response A: Correct. Nephelometry is a method using low angle forward scattering of an incident light source to measure the cloudiness or turbidity caused by aggregated immune complexes.

Learning Response B: Incorrect. 2% polyethylene glycol (PEG) alters the solubility of immune complexes causing them to precipitate out of solution.

Learning Response C: Incorrect. 50% ammonium sulfate alters the solubility of immune complexes causing them to precipitate out of solution.

Learning Response D: Incorrect. Anti-immunoglobulin will cross-link immune complexes and thus lead to their precipitation.

Learning Response E: Incorrect. The surface molecule protein A on Staphylococcal organisms binds to the Fc region of immunoglobulins, and the complex can then be spun down.

---

104. SUBJECT AREA: Core revision
QUESTION: Countercurrent immunoelectrophoresis is used to:

   A: Separate antigen from antibody
   B: Measure the affinity of an antibody
   C: Purify IgG antibodies
   D: Detect specific antibodies
   E: Separate antibodies with different isoelectric points

☐ Correct Answer: *D*

Learning Response A: Incorrect. In fact, in this technique the antibody and antigen are forced into contact with each other in order to form a line of precipitation.

Learning Response B: Incorrect. Countercurrent immunoelectrophoresis cannot be used to measure the affinity of an antibody.

Learning Response C: Incorrect. The technique is used for the detection, not purification, of antibodies.

Learning Response D: Correct. A rapid and fairly sensitive test which has been applied to the detection of antibodies to hepatitis B antigen, DNA antibodies in systemic lupus erythematosus (SLE), autoantibodies in mixed connective tissue disease and *Aspergillus* precipitins in cases with allergic bronchopulmonary aspergillosis.

Learning Response E: Incorrect. Antibodies can be separated in an electric field on the basis of differing isoelectric points, but the technique employed for this is called isoelectric focusing.

105. SUBJECT AREA: Estimation of antibody
QUESTION: The association constant (K_a) at equilibrium is represented by:

  A: [AgAb complex]
  B: [free Ag][free Ab]
  C: [free Ag][free Ab]/[AgAb complex]
  D: [AgAb complex]/[free Ag][free Ab]
  E: [free Ag]/[free Ab]

☐ Correct Answer: *D*

Learning Response A: Incorrect. Does not take into account the concentration of free antigen or free antibody, which must be included in any calculation of the association constant.

Learning Response B: Incorrect. Does not take into account the concentration of antigen-antibody complex, which must be included in any calculation of the association constant.

Learning Response C: Incorrect. This is the *dissociation* constant (K_d), not the association constant (K_a).

Learning Response D: Correct. This is the mass action equation at equilibrium, which provides a measure of the binding strength of an antibody for antigen, i.e., antibody affinity.

Learning Response E: Incorrect. Does not take into account the concentration of antigen-antibody complex, which must be included in any calculation of the association constant.

106.
SUBJECT AREA: Core revision
QUESTION: The affinity of an antibody can be determined by measuring:

- A: Its concentration
- B: The valency of antigen binding
- C: The amount of antibody bound at various antigen concentrations
- D: Its ability to neutralize bacterial toxins
- E: The sedimentation coefficient of the antibody

☐ Correct Answer: *C*

Learning Response A: Incorrect. This does not provide any information on the binding strength of the antibody.

Learning Response B: Incorrect. Although the valency will determine the avidity (functional affinity) of the antibody, it does not provide any information about the binding strength, i.e., intrinsic affinity, of each antibody arm.

Learning Response C: Correct. Affinity is measured by a variety of methods. Equilibrium dialysis is a useful method for haptens and other small molecules which are able to diffuse through dialysis tubing. For larger antigens other methods must be used, such as the ability of increasing amounts of unlabeled antigen to inhibit the binding of antibody to a radioactively labeled form of the same antigen.

Learning Response D: Incorrect. Although neutralization may well improve with increases in affinity of toxin-specific antibody, it does not provide a measure of the binding strength of the antibody. Note, however, that the 'bottom line' is how well the antibody performs functionally rather than the affinity per se.

Learning Response E: Incorrect. This provides no information regarding affinity, but does give a clue as to antibody valency, e.g., monomeric IgG has a sedimentation coefficient of 7 whereas pentameric IgM is 19.

---

107. SUBJECT AREA: Estimation of antibody
QUESTION: Latex particles are often used in:

      A: Agglutination tests
      B: Affinity chromatography
      C: Affinity measurements
      D: Adjuvants
      E: Neutralization assays

☐ Correct Answer: *A*

Learning Response A: Correct. In the past erythrocytes coated with antigen (e.g., thyroglobulin-coated turkey erythrocytes) have often been used in agglutination assays. Currently, latex particles are more frequently used as the solid phase onto which the antigen is coated.

Learning Response B: Incorrect. Sepharose, rather than latex, particles are normally employed in affinity chromatography.

Learning Response C: Incorrect. Although some assays for the measurement of affinity may utilize latex particles, the more commonly used methods do not.

Learning Response D: Incorrect. Adjuvants nonspecifically enhance immune responses to antigens. Latex particles do not have this property.

Learning Response E: Incorrect. Latex particles are not used in neutralization assays.

---

108. SUBJECT AREA: Estimation of antibody
QUESTION: The RAST measures:

      A: Antigen concentration
      B: IgE antibodies
      C: IgM antibodies
      D: Agglutination
      E: IgG antibodies

☐ Correct Answer: *B*

Learning Response A: Incorrect. It measures the amount of antibody, not antigen.

Learning Response B: Correct. The radioallergosorbent test (RAST) specifically measures IgE antibodies in allergic patients. The allergen, for example pollen extract, is covalently coupled to a paper disc which is then treated with patient's serum. The amount of specific IgE bound is determined using labeled anti-IgE.

Learning Response C: Incorrect. The RAST does measure a particular class of antibody, but not IgM.

Learning Response D: Incorrect. The RAST is not an agglutination assay.

Learning Response E: Incorrect. The RAST does measure a particular class of antibody, but not IgG.

109.
SUBJECT AREA: Core revision
QUESTION: In an ELISA you might use an antigen or antibody labeled with:

A: ^{125}I
B: FITC
C: Bentonite
D: Europium 3^+
E: Horseradish Peroxidase

☐ Correct Answer: *E*

Learning Response A: Incorrect. This would be a radioimmunoassay (RIA) as ^{125}I is a radioactive isotope of iodine. This label is employed in many immunoassays as can give good sensitivity and high signal:noise ratio.

Learning Response B: Incorrect. FITC (fluorescein isothiocyanate) is a fluorophore which emits green fluorescence when excited by UV light. An immunoassay using a ligand labeled with this reagent would therefore be termed an immunofluorescence (IF) assay, not an ELISA.

Learning Response C: Incorrect. Bentonite coated with antigen is sometimes used in agglutination assays for antibody detection.

Learning Response D: Incorrect. Time-resolved fluorescence uses a short excitation pulse and measures the signal after background has fallen to zero but before the Europium (which has a long fluorescence half-life) has decayed completely. This system permits good discrimination between a weak signal and background.

Learning Response E: Correct. Enzyme-linked immunosorbent assays (ELISA) use reagents that are labeled with enzymes which catalyse a color change in a substrate, e.g., horseradish peroxidase, alkaline phosphatase.

110.
SUBJECT AREA: Estimation of antibody
QUESTION: Surface plasmon resonance is a system based on:

- A: Fluorescence
- B: Radioactivity
- C: Reflected light
- D: Molecular resonance
- E: Magnetic fields

☐ Correct Answer: C

Learning Response A: Incorrect. When antibody-antigen binding is being measured these systems are called immunofluorescence.

Learning Response B: Incorrect. When antibody-antigen binding is being measured these systems are called radioimmunoassays.

Learning Response C: Correct. Monoclonal antibody is coupled to dextran which overlays a gold film on a glass prism sensor chip. Antigen present in a pulse of fluid will bind the sensor chip and, by increasing the amount of protein, will alter the angle of reflection of light. The system provides data on the kinetics of association and dissociation.

Learning Response D: Incorrect. Nuclear magnetic resonance (NMR) can provide structural information on molecules.

Learning Response E: Incorrect. Surface plasmon resonance is not based on magnetic fields.

111. SUBJECT AREA: Identification and measurement of antigens
QUESTION: The Ouchterlony double diffusion method relies on the reaction of antigen and antibody in (or on):

  A: Agar
  B: Streptavidin
  C: Gold-plated sensor chip
  D: Turkey erythrocytes
  E: Plastic microtiter plates

☐ Correct Answer: *A*

Learning Response A: Correct. Antigen and antibody are placed in wells cut in agar and diffuse towards each other. The precipitin reaction between antigen and antibody in the gel is detected as an opaque line in the region where they meet in optimal proportions.

Learning Response B: Incorrect. Streptavidin binds to biotin with extremely high affinity ($K = 10^{15}$ M^{-1}). Labeled streptavidin (for example, labeled with FITC or peroxidase) can therefore be used as a detection step for antibodies which have themselves been labeled with the vitamin biotin.

Learning Response C: Incorrect. Surface plasmon resonance, a technique that provides information on antibody association and dissociation rates ('on' and 'off' rates), utilizes antibody or antigen coupled to dextran overlaying a gold-plated sensor chip.

Learning Response D: Incorrect. The technique of hemagglutination is often carried out using turkey erythrocytes coated with antigen. Erythrocytes from this species are particularly suitable because antibodies to the turkey erythrocytes themselves are not commonly found in human subjects and they sediment rapidly. Nevertheless, a negative control of uncoated erythrocytes (or erythrocytes coated with an irrelevant antigen) must always be included in order to detect false positives.

Learning Response E: Incorrect. Plastic microtiter plates have many uses in immunological tests (e.g., solid phase radioimmunoassay, ELISA, agglutination, proliferation and cytotoxicity assays) but are not used in the Ouchterlony technique.

112. SUBJECT AREA: Identification and measurement of antigens
QUESTION: The presence of a 'spur' in the Ouchterlony test when two antigen samples are tested side by side indicates that they are:

- A: Identical
- B: Unrelated
- C: A mixture of antigens, one of which is identical, the others unrelated
- D: Partially related
- E: Able to recognize each other

☐ Correct Answer: *D*

Learning Response A: Incorrect. In this case the lines of precipitation would be completely confluent. Note, however, that the immunological identity is only in relation to the antiserum used and does not confirm molecular identity.

Learning Response B: Incorrect. In this instance the lines of precipitation would cross each other.

Learning Response C: Incorrect. In this case the lines of precipitation would cross each other for the unrelated antigens, and there would also be a completely confluent line representing the two identical antigens.

Learning Response D: Correct. A spur is formed when the antiserum used recognizes both an epitope shared between the two antigens and an epitope found only on one of the antigens.

Learning Response E: Incorrect. In the fairly unlikely event that the two antigens recognized each other, a precipitin line would form between the two antigen-containing wells and would cross the antigen-antibody precipitin line at right angles.

113. SUBJECT AREA: Identification and measurement of antigens
QUESTION: In single radial immunodiffusion, the antiserum is most commonly placed in:

- A: A well
- B: A trough
- C: Agar
- D: An electric field
- E: A tube

☐ Correct Answer: *C*

Learning Response A: Incorrect. Although the technique can be employed using antiserum placed in a well, it is the antigen that is normally placed in the well in single radial immunodiffusion (SRI).

Learning Response B: Incorrect. This is normally the case in immuno-electrophoresis.

Learning Response C: Correct. The test sample is placed in a well and allowed to diffuse into the antibody-containing gel. The diameter of the precipitin ring can be used to give a quantitative measure of the amount of antigen if it is compared to a calibration curve produced using known amounts of antigen.

Learning Response D: Incorrect. The technique does not employ electrophoresis but relies on the diffusion of antigen into the gel.

Learning Response E: Incorrect. In single radial immunodiffusion the antiserum is not placed in a tube.

114.
SUBJECT AREA: Identification and measurement of antigens
QUESTION: Western blots are primarily used to detect:

A: Protein
B: Carbohydrate
C: Lipid
D: RNA
E: DNA

☐ Correct Answer: *A*

Learning Response A: Correct. Following separation by techniques such as SDS-PAGE or isoelectric focusing, proteins can be blotted by transverse electrophoresis onto nitrocellulose membranes and can then be identified by staining with appropriately labeled antibodies.

Learning Response B: Incorrect. However, carbohydrates attached to the molecules which are normally analysed by Western blotting may be detectable using lectins or antibodies specific for particular sugars.

Learning Response C: Incorrect. Lipids are not analysed using Western blotting.

Learning Response D: Incorrect. The transfer of RNA from electrophoresis gels to nitrocellulose or nylon membranes is called Northern blotting.

Learning Response E: Incorrect. The transfer of DNA from electrophoresis gels to nitrocellulose or nylon membranes is called Southern blotting.

115. SUBJECT AREA: Identification and measurement of antigens
QUESTION: SDS-PAGE separates proteins on the basis of:

        A: Isoelectric point
        B: Sedimentation coefficient
        C: Amino acid sequence
        D: Degree of glycosylation
        E: Size

☐ Correct Answer: *E*

Learning Response A: Incorrect. Proteins can be separated on the basis of their isoelectric point using isoelectric focusing, not SDS-PAGE.

Learning Response B: Incorrect. Centrifugation techniques are used to separate proteins on the basis of their sedimentation coefficient.

Learning Response C: Incorrect. Amino acid sequence, together with glycosylation, will determine the overall charge and the isoelectric point of the protein, criteria which can be used to separate proteins using normal electrophoresis or ion exchange chromatography on the one hand and isoelectric focusing on the other.

Learning Response D: Incorrect. The degree of glycosylation does affect the migration of proteins on SDS-PAGE, but this technique is not conventionally used to separate proteins on the basis of their degree of glycosylation.

Learning Response E: Correct. Although SDS-PAGE separates proteins of different sizes, the separation itself is based upon charge. The larger the molecule the more sodium dodecyl sulfate (SDS) it will bind and therefore the more negatively charged it will be. Thus proteins of different sizes can be separated by electrophoresis in a gel such as polyacrylamide on the basis of overall charge. By running molecular weight markers at the same time, an approximate molecular weight can be estimated.

116. SUBJECT AREA: Identification and measurement of antigens
QUESTION: The pepscan technique is most useful for determining:

        A: Antibody structure
        B: Discontinuous epitopes recognized by antibodies
        C: Epitopes recognized by T cells
        D: MHC haplotypes
        E: TCR Vβ usage

☐ Correct Answer: *C*

Learning Response A: Incorrect. This technique does not provide information related to antibody structure, although it can be used to delineate linear epitopes on antibody molecules.

Learning Response B: Incorrect. Although the techique is useful for detecting linear (continuous) determinants, most epitopes recognized by antibodies are discontinuous and these cannot be fully detected using the pepscan technique.

Learning Response C: Correct. Cleavable peptides synthesized on pins provide molecules which can be used to determine epitopes which will bind to MHC molecules and be presented to the T-cell receptor.

Learning Response D: Incorrect. Cleavable peptides synthesized on pins can provide molecules which can be used to determine epitopes which will bind to MHC molecules of different haplotypes, but this would be an extremely laborious approach for determining an MHC haplotype.

Learning Response E: Incorrect. Cleavable peptides synthesized on pins can provide molecules which can be used to determine epitopes which will bind to MHC molecules and be presented to T-cell receptors bearing different Vβ segments, but antibodies to specific Vβs are usually used as a much simpler approach.

117. SUBJECT AREA: Making antibodies to order
QUESTION: HAT medium is used to:

        A: Immortalize B lymphocytes
        B: Culture B lymphocytes
        C: Select for hybrids in the hybridoma technique
        D: Kill B cell hybridomas
        E: Fuse B lymphocytes to myeloma cells

☐ Correct Answer: *C*

Learning Response A: Incorrect. B lymphocytes are killed by HAT medium.

Learning Response B: Incorrect. B lymphocytes are killed by HAT medium.

Learning Response C: Correct. HAT medium contains hypoxanthine, aminopterin and thymidine. Aminopterin blocks the principle pathway of DNA synthesis. An alternative ('salvage') pathway exists which utilizes hypoxanthine and thymidine. The tumor cell lines used for hybridoma production are mutants lacking the enzyme necessary for this pathway. Therefore, unfused tumor cells will die in HAT. Normal cells die because they are not immortal. However, the hybrids survive because they have the immortality of the tumor parent and the salvage pathway enzymes inherited from the normal B cells.

Learning Response D: Incorrect. B cell hybridomas are not killed in HAT medium.

Learning Response E: Incorrect. This can be achieved by several different methods, most commonly using polyethylene glycol.

118. SUBJECT AREA: Core revision
QUESTION: An abzyme is:

    A: An enzyme used to digest antibody
    B: An immunoadsorbent
    C: Found in the vacuoles of phagocytic cells
    D: An antibody that is capable of acting as an enzyme
    E: An antibody to zymosan

☐ Correct Answer: *D*

Learning Response A: Incorrect. Proteolytic enzymes such as papain or pepsin can be used to produce antibody fragments (Fab and $F(ab')_2$, respectively).

Learning Response B: Incorrect. An abzyme is not an immunoadsorbent.

Learning Response C: Incorrect. Enzymes such as lysozyme, together with various hydrolytic enzymes, are present in the vacuoles of phagocytic cells.

Learning Response D: Correct. Abzymes are sometimes referred to as catalytic antibodies. These monoclonal antibodies to stable analogues of the transition state of a given reaction can act as an enzyme ('abzyme') in catalyzing that reaction. Some abzymes have been described which catalyze reactions which are otherwise difficult to achieve.

Learning Response E: Incorrect. Zymosan is a component of yeast cell walls which acts as a powerful activator of phagocytic cells.

---

119. SUBJECT AREA: Making antibodies to order
QUESTION: A single chain Fv fragment (scFv) will:

- *A:* Fix C1q
- *B:* Bear idiotypes
- *C:* Cross-link antigen
- *D:* Only be present on the surface of filamentous bacteriophage
- *E:* Possess either V_H or V_L but not both

☐ Correct Answer: *B*

Learning Response A: Incorrect. This is a function of the constant region of the immunoglobulin heavy chain.

Learning Response B: Correct. Idiotypes are variable region-associated antigenic determinants.

Learning Response C: Incorrect. A single chain Fv (scFv) is monovalent and therefore unable to cross-link antigen.

Learning Response D: Incorrect. Although a scFv can be expressed on the surface of filamentous phage, they can also be produced in soluble form.

Learning Response E: Incorrect. A conventional scFv consists of a V_H domain linked to a V_L domain by a flexible linker peptide.

---

120. SUBJECT AREA: Purification of antigens and antibodies by affinity chromatography
QUESTION: In affinity chromatography the required ligand is often released by:

- *A:* Changing the pH
- *B:* Vigorous shaking
- *C:* Changing the temperature from 37° to 4°C

D: Boiling
E: Adding a small amount of detergent (e.g., 0.025% Tween 20)

☐ Correct Answer: A

Learning Response A: Correct. Antigen-antibody bonds can be disrupted by changing the pH or adding chaotropic agents such as thiocyanate.

Learning Response B: Incorrect. Although antigen-antibody bonds are noncovalent, they are not disrupted so easily by such sheer forces.

Learning Response C: Incorrect. This would not lead to release of the ligand but would probably increase avidity.

Learning Response D: Incorrect. This might release the ligand but the protein structure would be destroyed and therefore this is not usually an option.

Learning Response E: Incorrect. Antibody-antigen bonds are not disrupted in this low level of detergent. In fact, 0.025% Tween 20 is often used in antibody-binding assays to reduce nonspecific interactions whilst allowing specific binding to occur.

121. SUBJECT AREA: Isolation of leukocyte subpopulations
QUESTION: Coating a cell with specific antibody facilitates its selection by:

A: Sedimentation rate
B: Buoyant density
C: Adherence to plastic surfaces
D: Magnetic beads coated with anti-Ig
E: Light scatter in the fluorescence activated cell sorter (FACS)

☐ Correct Answer: D

Learning Response A: Incorrect. Sedimentation rate separates cells on the basis of size.

Learning Response B: Incorrect. Buoyant density separates cells on the basis of their density.

Learning Response C: Incorrect. Coating with antibody does not significantly affect the adherence to plastic. This is a feature of phagocytic cells and to a much lesser extent, B cells.

Learning Response D: Correct. The magnetic beads coated with anti-immunoglobulin will bind to the cells which are coated on their surface with antibody and can be separated with a magnet.

Learning Response E: Incorrect. Light scatter in the FACS can be used in the forward mode to give information on cell size and in the 90° scatter mode, to give information on cell granularity.

---

122. SUBJECT AREA: Isolation of leukocyte subpopulations
QUESTION: A T cell hybridoma:

- *A:* Is obtained by stimulating T cells with antigen
- *B:* Is obtained by cloning antigen-specific splenic T cells
- *C:* Is obtained by fusing T cells with a T-cell tumor cell line and cloning
- *D:* Expresses a multiplicity of T-cell receptor specificities
- *E:* Results from introducing transgenes for the rearranged α- and β-receptor from a T-cell clone

☐ Correct Answer: *C*

Learning Response A: Incorrect. Continually stimulating sensitized T cells with the antigen will lead to proliferation of a *T-cell line,* which is a polyclonal mixture of T cells with different fine specificities for the antigen.

Learning Response B: Incorrect. The cloning will produce T cells of a single specificity but they will not divide spontaneously as does a T cell hybridoma, but only under the influence of further contact with antigen.

Learning Response C: Correct. The specificity of the T cell hybridoma clones will be married to the immortality of the T-cell tumor cell line. Thus we have a spontaneously dividing antigen specific T-cell clone.

Learning Response D: Incorrect. A T-cell hybridoma represents a clone with a single receptor specificity.

Learning Response E: Incorrect. Introducing transgenes for rearranged T-cell receptors will prevent all T cells from any further rearrangement of β-receptors although not of another α-receptor. Therefore virtually all the T cells will include the specificity of the original transgenes. However, these will be normal T cells in their responses to antigen and will not have the uncontrolled cell division of a T cell hybridoma.

123. SUBJECT AREA: Immunohistochemistry
QUESTION: Which of the following is *not* used as a direct conjugate to the antibody for visualizing tissue antigen:

    A: Fluorescein
    B: Anti-immunoglobulin
    C: Alkaline phosphatase
    D: ^{131}I
    E: Gold particles

☐ Correct Answer: *B*

Learning Response A: Incorrect. Fluorescein conjugates are visualized in the fluorescence microscope.

Learning Response B: Correct. Anti-immunoglobulin is used to detect the binding of antibody to tissue antigens, but can only be visualized by conjugation with an appropriate molecule.

Learning Response C: Incorrect. Alkaline phosphatase conjugates are visualized by colour reactions.

Learning Response D: Incorrect. The radioactive iodine conjugates can be detected by autoradiography.

Learning Response E: Incorrect. The gold particles are detectable in the electron microscope.

124. SUBJECT AREA: Immunohistochemistry
QUESTION: A confocal microscope at high magnification does *not*:

    A: Bring all focal planes of an image into focus simultaneously
    B: Permit construction of a 3-dimensional image
    C: Improve the quality of image definition in a single plane
    D: Provide quantitative data
    E: Function with fluorescent conjugates

☐ Correct Answer: *A*

Learning Response A: Correct. The microscope focuses on a single focal plane.

Learning Response B: Incorrect. 3-D images can be constructed from the computer images recorded at each focal plane.

Learning Response C: Incorrect. The image definition in the single plane is enhanced in quality because the other planes which are out of focus and therefore fuzzy, are eliminated from the image.

Learning Response D: Incorrect.

Learning Response E: Incorrect.

---

125. SUBJECT AREA: Immunohistochemistry
QUESTION: The use of propidium iodide in flow cytofluorimetry permits measurement of:

- *A:* Cell size
- *B:* Cell granularity
- *C:* Cell surface antigens
- *D:* Apoptosis
- *E:* Intracellular gene expression

☐ Correct Answer: *D*

Learning Response A: Incorrect. Cell size is computed from forward light scatter.

Learning Response B: Incorrect. Granularity is computed from 90° light scatter.

Learning Response C: Incorrect. Cell surface antigens are recognized by fluorescent conjugates of antibodies.

Learning Response D: Correct. Propidium iodide binds to intracellular DNA and gives a quantitative measurement. In apoptotic cells, the DNA which is broken down gives cells with less than the diploid level.

Learning Response E: Incorrect. Gene expression must be coupled to a reporter gene whose expression leads to the creation of an intracellular fluorescent product.

126. SUBJECT AREA: Assessment of functional activity
QUESTION: The activation of lymphocytes *cannot* be assessed by:

    A: Mitosis
    B: Cytokine release
    C: Phagocytosis
    D: Cytotoxicity
    E: Limiting dilution analysis

☐ Correct Answer: *C*

Learning Response A: Incorrect. On activation, lymphocytes are pushed into the cell cycle.

Learning Response B: Incorrect. On activation, cytokine genes become derepressed.

Learning Response C: Correct. Lymphocytes are not phagocytic, irrespective of their activation status.

Learning Response D: Incorrect. Lymphocytes for the appropriate subset can become cytotoxic for other cells on activation.

Learning Response E: Incorrect. Limiting dilution analysis provides an estimate of the number of lymphocytes which become activated. At a dilution of the lymphocyte population at which 37% of wells give a negative response, each well on average will contain one precursor lymphocyte.

127. SUBJECT AREA: Assessment of functional activity
QUESTION: Antibody forming cells can be enumerated by:

    A: Mitosis
    B: Cytokine release
    C: Total antibody content
    D: Cell surface immunoglobulin
    E: Plaque techniques

☐ Correct Answer: *E*

Learning Response A: Incorrect. Cell division is not related to the formation of antibody.

Learning Response B: Incorrect. Cytokine release is unrelated to antibody formation.

Learning Response C: Incorrect. Total antibody content cannot be used to calculate the number of antibody forming cells since they each may synthesize and secrete different amounts of antibody.

Learning Response D: Incorrect. Cell surface immunoglobulin is unrelated to antibody synthesis and indeed the terminal plasma cell has very little if any surface Ig.

Learning Response E: Correct. Each antibody forming cell can be caused to form an individual plaque so allowing enumeration.

---

128. SUBJECT AREA: Genetic engineering of cells
QUESTION: Introduction of a gene into a cell using calcium phosphate precipitate is termed:

- *A:* Electroporation
- *B:* Homologous recombination
- *C:* Biolistics
- *D:* Transfection
- *E:* Mutation

☐ Correct Answer: *D*

Learning Response A: Incorrect. Electroporation is a means of introducing a gene into a cell by a brief electric pulse.

Learning Response B: Incorrect. This is a situation in which a disrupted gene fragment can replace the resident normal gene.

Learning Response C: Incorrect. Genes can be introduced into cells by firing them at high speed coated onto gold microparticles.

Learning Response D: Correct. Transfection is the introduction of a gene into a cell; calcium phosphate precipitate is one method of achieving this.

Learning Response E: Incorrect. Mutation involves change in the DNA sequence of a gene.

129.
SUBJECT AREA: Core revision
QUESTION: Antigen-specific B cells can be purified by:

- A: Sedimentation rate
- B: Panning on anti-Ig plates
- C: Phagocytosis
- D: Forward light scatter in the fluorescence activated cell sorter (FACS)
- E: Binding of fluorescent antigen and separation in the FACS

☐ Correct Answer: *E*

Learning Response A: Incorrect. Sedimentation rate separates cells on the basis of size and so would enrich small lymphocytes if required but would not purify the antigen-specific B cells.

Learning Response B: Incorrect. B cells with surface Ig would adhere to anti-Ig plates but there would be no selection of the antigen-specific B cells.

Learning Response C: Incorrect. B cells are not essentially phagocytic.

Learning Response D: Incorrect. Forward light scatter in the FACS separates cells on the basis of their size not antigen specificity.

Learning Response E: Correct. Antigen-specific B cells would specifically bind the fluorescent antigen and provide a signal in the FACS which would be utilized to select these cells.

130.
SUBJECT AREA: Core revision
QUESTION: Antigens in tissues can be localized with fluorescent antibodies using:

- A: Flow cytofluorimetry
- B: A confocal fluorescence microscope
- C: Autoradiography
- D: An enzyme substrate
- E: The electron microscope

☐ Correct Answer: *B*

Learning Response A: Incorrect. Flow cytofluorimetry requires analysis of a cell suspension not a tissue.

Learning Response B: Correct. The confocal fluorescence microscope will clearly define the localization of antigens in tissues which have bound fluorescent antibody and the optics enable high resolution at high magnification.

Learning Response C: Incorrect. Autoradiography utilizes the radiation from radiolabeled conjugates not fluorescent conjugates, and this is picked up on photograph film as an autoradiograph.

Learning Response D: Incorrect. Fluorescent antibodies do not per se act on enzyme substrates although enzyme conjugates of antibodies can be used in this way to give a coloured reaction product.

Learning Response E: Incorrect. Fluorescent antibodies do not show up in the EM. One would use gold particles of different sizes with the antibodies attached to their surface.

131. SUBJECT AREA: Core revision
QUESTION: The functional activity of polymorphs (neutrophils) can be assessed by:

A: The nitroblue tetrazolium test
B: Proliferation
C: Limiting dilution analysis
D: A plaque test for antibody
E: A fluorescent antibody test for myeloperoxidase

☐ Correct Answer: *A*

Learning Response A: Correct. Phagocytosis activates the NADPH oxidase which converts the nitroblue tetrazolium salt through electron transfer into a blue formazan.

Learning Response B: Incorrect. Polys do not proliferate.

Learning Response C: Incorrect. Limiting dilution analysis is a means for establishing the frequency of a given cell type or its precursor. It is not a measure of functional activity.

Learning Response D: Incorrect. Polymorphs do not secrete antibody. The plaque test is utilized for antibody secreting cells such as plasma cells.

Learning Response E: Incorrect. The fluorescent antibody test for myeloperoxidase will pick out the polymorphs and macrophages, but not give an estimate of their functional activity.

132. SUBJECT AREA: Core revision
QUESTION: A gene can be selectively disrupted by:

   A: Electroporation
   B: Homologous recombination
   C: Liposome transfection
   D: Antisense RNA
   E: X-Irradiation

☐ Correct Answer: *B*

Learning Response A: Incorrect. Electroporation is a means of transfecting a cell by introducing a gene. Only if the gene is of a special nature can one disrupt the native gene by homologous recombination.

Learning Response B: Correct. Homologous recombination is a relatively rare event which involves interchange of a transfected genetic sequence with that of the homologous native gene and if one introduces an alteration in the reading frame, this will selectively disrupt gene expression.

Learning Response C: Incorrect. Liposome transfection is a means of introducing genes into a cell. Only if the gene is of a particular nature will it disrupt by homologous recombination.

Learning Response D: Incorrect. Antisense RNA introduced into a cell will base-pair with target mRNA and block translation into protein.

Learning Response E: Incorrect. X-irradiation provides random damage rather than selective disruption of genes.

133. SUBJECT AREA: The need for organized lymphoid tissue
QUESTION: Which one of the following is a primary lymphoid organ:

   A: Lymph nodes
   B: Spleen
   C: Peyer's patch
   D: Tonsil
   E: Thymus

☐ Correct Answer: *E*

Learning Response A: Incorrect. The lymph nodes occur at the junctions of the lymphatic vessels and essentially filter off and respond to foreign material draining from the tissues. They form part of the peripheral, or secondary, lymphoid tissue.

Learning Response B: Incorrect. The spleen monitors the blood and removes effete red and white cells as well as responding to blood-borne antigens. The spleen forms part of the peripheral, or secondary, lymphoid tissue, although in the fetus it acts as a primary lymphoid organ.

Learning Response C: Incorrect. The Peyer's patches are unencapsulated mucosal-associated lymphoid tissues in the small intestine. Antigen enters across specialized epithelial cells and stimulates cells committed to IgA and IgE synthesis.

Learning Response D: Incorrect. The tonsils, together with the adenoids and associated lymph nodes, form the Waldeyer's ring of lymphoid tissue.

Learning Response E: Correct. The secondary lymphoid tissues become populated by macrophages and lymphocytes derived from bone marrow stem cells and by T cells which first differentiate into immunocompetent cells in the thymus.

---

134. SUBJECT AREA: Core revision
QUESTION: The spleen is largely involved with the response to antigens which are in the:

A: Tissues
B: Blood
C: Gut
D: Lungs
E: Urogenital tract

☐ Correct Answer: *B*

Learning Response A: Incorrect. Draining lymph nodes at the junctions of lymphatic vessels deal with antigens derived from the tissues.

Learning Response B: Correct. The spleen can be thought of as a filter sampling the blood for effete red cells and for foreign antigens.

Learning Response C: Incorrect. The mucosal-associated lymphoid tissues (MALT) are concerned with responding to antigens in the gut, largely by mounting IgA or IgE responses.

Learning Response D: Incorrect. The bronchus-associated lymphoid tissue (BALT) provides protective IgA responses against antigen entering the airways.

Learning Response E: Incorrect. The mucosal-associated lymphoid tissues (MALT) produce protective IgA responses in the urogenital tract.

135. SUBJECT AREA: The need for organized lymphoid tissue
QUESTION: The thoracic duct:

- *A:* Enters the spleen
- *B:* Directly drains the lymph nodes
- *C:* Forms the interface between the lymph and blood
- *D:* Transports T cells from the bone marrow to the thymus
- *E:* Is a part of the lamina propria

☐ Correct Answer: *C*

Learning Response A: Incorrect. The spleen is a highly vascularized secondary lymphoid organ into which blood enters via the splenic artery. It is a very effective blood filter removing effete red and white blood cells and responding actively to blood-borne antigens.

Learning Response B: Incorrect. The efferent lymphatics drain the lymph nodes.

Learning Response C: Correct. The lymphatics and associated lymph nodes form a network draining the viscera and the more superficial body structures before returning to the blood by way of the thoracic duct.

Learning Response D: Incorrect. Lymphocytes that are destined to become T cells pass from the bone marrow to the thymus via blood vessels. This process is controlled by 'homing' adhesion molecules.

Learning Response E: Incorrect. The lamina propria is unencapsulated lymphoid tissue underlying the gut wall.

136. SUBJECT AREA: Lymphocytes traffic between lymphoid tissues
QUESTION: When antigen reaches a lymph node in a primed animal:

A: There is an increase in the output of cells in the efferent lymphatics over the following 24 hours
B: There is a decrease in the output of cells in the efferent lymphatics over the following 24 hours
C: There is an immediate output of activated blast cells
D: It is transported to the spleen
E: It is all immediately destroyed by macrophages

☐ Correct Answer: *B*

Learning Response A: Incorrect. There is no increase in the output of cells in the efferent lymphatics over the 24 hours following the arrival of antigen at a lymph node in a primed animal.

Learning Response B: Correct. Antigen-reactive cells are depleted from the circulating pool of lymphocytes within 24 hours of antigen first localizing in the lymph nodes or spleen, and there is a dramatic fall in the output of cells in the efferent lymphatics.

Learning Response C: Incorrect. A peak of activated blast cell output occurs at around 80 hours following the arrival of antigen at a lymph node.

Learning Response D: Incorrect. Generally, tissue-derived antigens are dealt with by the draining lymph nodes whilst blood-borne antigens elicit immune responses in the spleen.

Learning Response E: Incorrect. Although macrophages are able to degrade phagocytosed antigen very efficiently, at least a proportion of the antigen remains for long periods of time as immune complexes on the surface of follicular dendritic cells, which are thought to be involved in the generation of memory B cells.

137. SUBJECT AREA: Lymphocytes traffic between lymphoid tissues
QUESTION: The specialized cell type involved in the entry of lymphocytes into lymph nodes are called:

A: M cells
B: Mesangial cells
C: PALS
D: HEV
E: Selectins

☐ Correct Answer: *D*

Learning Response A: Incorrect. Antigen is largely excluded from entering the body by the mucosal epithelial cells which have tight junctions and a protective mucus layer. However, specialized antigen-transporting M cells interspersed between the gut columnar epithelium pass antigen from the gut to the underlying antigen-presenting cells.

Learning Response B: Incorrect. Mesangial cells are the phagocytic macrophages of the kidney.

Learning Response C: Incorrect. The PALS is a tissue, not a cell. These *periarteriolar lymphoid sheaths* in the spleen consist predominantly of T cells which surround the splenic arterioles.

Learning Response D: Correct. The high-walled endothelium of the post-capillary venules (HEV) in lymph nodes express vascular addressins which are recognized by homing receptors on lymphocytes passing through the afferent lymphatics and which mediate entry of the lymphocytes into the lymph nodes.

Learning Response E: Incorrect. Selectins are a family of molecules, not cells. L-selectin is involved in entry of lymphocytes into lymph nodes and is the lymphocyte homing receptor which recognizes the high endothelial venule (HEV) addressin molecule.

---

138. SUBJECT AREA: Core revision
QUESTION: The germinal center is an important site of:

  A: Hematopoiesis
  B: B-cell maturation
  C: T-cell maturation
  D: Myeloid cell differentiation
  E: Germ line V gene rearrangement

☐ Correct Answer: *B*

Learning Response A: Incorrect. In the adult, hematopoiesis occurs in the bone marrow.

Learning Response B: Correct. The germinal center contains large, usually proliferating, B-blasts. They are important sites of maturation to antibody producing cells and for the generation of B cell memory and are therefore greatly enlarged during secondary antibody responses.

Learning Response C: Incorrect. Germinal centers contain relatively small numbers of T cells, the majority of these being confined to the paracortical (thymus-dependent) area of the lymph node.

Learning Response D: Incorrect. Although there are scattered macrophages present in germinal centers, it is not a site of myeloid cell differentiation.

Learning Response E: Incorrect. B cells will have already rearranged their germ line V genes by the time they appear in germinal centers. However, rearrangement of constant region genes will occur during immunoglobulin class switching from IgM^+ IgD^+ to other isotypes; a major feature of the germinal center.

139. SUBJECT AREA: Encapsulated lymph nodes
QUESTION: The tingible bodies inside germinal center macrophages are:

- *A:* DNA fragments
- *B:* Phagocytosed foreign antigen
- *C:* A sign of macrophage apoptosis
- *D:* Bacterial cell wall components resistant to degradation
- *E:* VLA molecules

☐ Correct Answer: *A*

Learning Response A: Correct. There is very extensive apoptotic cell death amongst light zone centrocytes and the resultant DNA fragments are visible as 'tingible bodies' within the macrophages which have phagocytosed the apoptotic lymphocytes.

Learning Response B: Incorrect. Germinal center macrophages do phagocytose external antigen, but this is not the origin of the tingible bodies.

Learning Response C: Incorrect. They are not a sign of macrophage apoptosis.

Learning Response D: Incorrect. Bacterial cell walls are not the source of the tingible bodies.

Learning Response E: Incorrect. VLA molecules are widely distributed integrins involved in adhesion to ligands such as laminin, collagen and fibronectin.

140. SUBJECT AREA: Encapsulated lymph nodes
QUESTION: The paracortical area of a lymph node comprises mainly:

- *A:* Follicular dendritic cells
- *B:* Plasma cells

C: Macrophages
D: B cells
E: T cells

☐ Correct Answer: *E*

Learning Response A: Incorrect. Follicular dendritic cells are found in primary and secondary follicles of lymph nodes, and in the germinal centers they form a tight network of cells with elongated cytoplasmic processes.

Learning Response B: Incorrect. The plasma cells are mainly found in the medullary cords which project between the medullary sinuses, a site distinct from that at which antigen triggering has occurred. This may prevent the generation of high local concentrations of antibody within the germinal center to avoid neutralization of the antigen on the follicular dendritic cells.

Learning Response C: Incorrect. Macrophages are scattered throughout the lymph nodes but are found especially in the medullary sinuses and in the basal light zone of the germinal centers.

Learning Response D: Incorrect. B cells are mostly located in the outer cortex.

Learning Response E: Correct. T cells are mainly confined to the paracortical (thymus-dependent) area of lymph nodes, and in nodes taken from children with selective T-cell deficiency the paracortical region is virtually devoid of lymphocytes.

141. SUBJECT AREA: Core revision
QUESTION: Lymphocytes in the lamina propria secrete large amounts of:

A: IgD
B: IgA
C: γδ TCR
D: Bence Jones protein
E: Isolated secretory component

☐ Correct Answer: *B*

Learning Response A: Incorrect. IgD is largely a cell-surface associated molecule which, together with IgM, acts as the antigen receptor on virgin B cells.

Learning Response B: Correct. In the gut, antigen enters Peyer's patches across specialized epithelial cells and stimulates antigen-sensitive lymphocytes which after activation drain into the lymph, then pass via the mesenteric lymph nodes, thoracic duct and blood stream, to the lamina propria where they become IgA-forming cells.

Learning Response C: Incorrect. In the mouse, but not in man, intraepithelial lymphocytes are predominantly T cells with the γδ T-cell receptor and may be specialized for the recognition of highly conserved microbial antigens such as heat-shock proteins. They perhaps act as a relatively primitive first line of defense at the outer surfaces of the body.

Learning Response D: Incorrect. Bence Jones proteins are isolated light chains found in the serum and urine of myeloma patients.

Learning Response E: Incorrect. Secretory component is a proteolytic cleavage product of the poly-Ig receptor which transports IgA from the lamina propria across the epithelia into the gut lumen. Therefore, secretory component is associated with the IgA and is not usually found in a free form.

142. SUBJECT AREA: Core revision
QUESTION: The bone marrow is a site of:

- A: Very little antibody production
- B: Antibody production against T-independent antigens only
- C: A major site of long term antibody production
- D: A major site of IgD secretion
- E: Antibody production by pre-B cells

☐ Correct Answer: *C*

Learning Response A: Incorrect. Antibody is produced in the bone marrow.

Learning Response B: Incorrect. Antibody against both T-dependent and T-independent antigens can be produced by B cells in the bone marrow.

Learning Response C: Correct. Bone marrow constitutes up to 80% of the total immunoglobulin-secreting cells in mice.

Learning Response D: Incorrect. IgD is not secreted in large amounts but is mainly a cell surface-associated immunoglobulin.

Learning Response E: Incorrect. Pre-B cells are immature and therefore are unable to secrete antbody. They possess intracytoplasmic μ heavy chain but lack surface immunoglobulin.

143. SUBJECT AREA: Core revision
QUESTION: An example of a privileged immunological site is the:

　　　　A: Bone marrow
　　　　B: Skin
　　　　C: Testis
　　　　D: Lung
　　　　E: Waldeyer's ring

☐ Correct Answer: C

Learning Response A: Incorrect. The bone marrow is rich in immunocompetent cells.

Learning Response B: Incorrect. Langerhans' cells in the skin pick up and process antigen, then travel as veiled cells in the lymph before becoming interdigitating dendritic cells in the paracortical T-cell zone of the draining lymph node where they are potent stimulators of T-cell responses.

Learning Response C: Correct. The brain, anterior chamber of the eye and the testis are privileged sites in which antigens are safely sequestered from the immune system by virtue of strong blood-tissue barriers and low permeability to hydrophilic compounds and carrier-mediated transport systems.

Learning Response D: Incorrect. IgA-forming cells are present in the bronchus-associated lymphoid tissue (BALT), a part of the secretory immune system which bathes mucosal surfaces with protective IgA antibodies.

Learning Response E: Incorrect. Lymph node, tonsil and adenoids provide protection against infectious agents present in the upper respiratory and alimentary tracts.

144. SUBJECT AREA: The handling of antigen
QUESTION: Langerhans' cells are found in:

　　　　　A: Lymph
　　　　　B: Lymph nodes
　　　　　C: Periarteriolar lymphoid sheaths
　　　　　D: Skin
　　　　　E: Mantle zone

☐ Correct Answer: *D*

Learning Response A: Incorrect. However, the veiled cells found in lymph are derived from Langerhans' cells.

Learning Response B: Incorrect. Langerhans' cells migrate to lymph nodes where they become interdigitating dendritic cells which initiate primary T-cell responses.

Learning Response C: Incorrect. The periarteriolar lymphoid sheaths (PALS) are T-cell areas of the spleen.

Learning Response D: Correct. Langerhans' cells in the skin pick up and process antigen, then travel as veiled cells in the lymph before becoming interdigitating dendritic cells in the paracortical T-cell zone of the draining lymph node, where they are potent stimulators of T-cell responses.

Learning Response E: Incorrect. The mantle zone of B lymphocytes surrounds the germinal center which together form a secondary follicle.

145. SUBJECT AREA: The handling of antigen
QUESTION: Which of the following functions are macrophages unable to carry out:

- *A:* Pinocytosis
- *B:* Phagocytosis
- *C:* Antigen processing
- *D:* T-cell priming
- *E:* Antigen presentation to activated cells

☐ Correct Answer: *D*

Learning Response A: Incorrect. Macrophages are extremely efficient at pinocytosis.

Learning Response B: Incorrect. Antigens are readily phagocytosed by macrophages, especially if first opsonized by coating with antibody and/or complement.

Learning Response C: Incorrect. Antigens taken up by macrophages are broken down in the lysosomes and can then be presented to T cells as processed peptide associated with MHC class II which is expressed on the macrophage following activation by bacterial components such as lipopolysaccharide (LPS).

Learning Response D: Correct. Macrophages have an impressive range of functions but appear unable to prime naive lymphocytes. This can be carried out by lymphoid interdigitating dendritic cells and cultured, but not freshly isolated, Langerhans' cells.

Learning Response E: Incorrect. Macrophages function as general antigen-presenting cells for primed lymphocytes.

146. SUBJECT AREA: Core revision
QUESTION: Follicular dendritic cells:

  A: Can bind immune complexes
  B: Are small round cells
  C: Retain antigen for up to 24 hours
  D: Possess Fc receptors but lack C3b receptors
  E: Are not found in germinal centers

☐ Correct Answer: *A*

Learning Response A: Correct. Secondary antibody responses can be boosted by quite small amounts of immunogen which complex with circulating antibody and fix C3 so that they localize very effectively on the surface of follicular dendritic cells within the germinal centers of secondary follicles.

Learning Response B: Incorrect. Follicular dendritic cells have very elongated processes which can make contact with numerous lymphocytes.

Learning Response C: Incorrect. Antigen can be detected on the surface of follicular dendritic cells for long periods of time and provide a sustained source of antigenic stimulation for the generation and maintenance of memory B cells.

Learning Response D: Incorrect. Follicular dendritic cells possess surface receptors for IgG Fc and for iC3b.

Learning Response E: Incorrect. Germinal centers possess a meshwork of follicular dendritic cells which expand B cell blasts produced by secondary antigen challenge, and direct their differentiation into memory cells and antibody-forming plasma cells.

147. SUBJECT AREA: Core revision
QUESTION: Lymphocytes:

> *A:* Enter the tissues and remain there for the rest of their life
> *B:* When mature are only found in secondary lymphoid organs
> *C:* Recirculate between blood and lymphoid tissues
> *D:* Are only educated in the thymus
> *E:* When present in the lymph are called veiled cells

☐ Correct Answer: *C*

Learning Response A: Incorrect. However, blood monocytes differentiate into macrophages upon entering the tissues and are thought to remain there for the rest of their life, as do granulocytes which enter the tissues from the circulation although they have a very short life in contrast.

Learning Response B: Incorrect. Mature lymphocytes are also found in the primary lymphoid organs. In fact, the bone marrow is a major site of antibody production by fully differentiated plasma cells.

Learning Response C: Correct. Lymphocyte recirculation between the blood and lymphoid tissues is guided by specialized homing receptors on the surface of high walled endothelium of the postcapillary venules. They then re-enter the bloodstream via the thoracic duct.

Learning Response D: Incorrect. Although T lymphocytes are educated in the thymus, B-lymphocyte education occurs in the bone marrow.

Learning Response E: Incorrect. The veiled cells in the lymph are derived from skin Langerhans' cells which are in the process of carrying antigen to the local lymph nodes where, as interdigitating dendritic cells (IDC) they settle down in the paracortical T-cell zone where they stimulate naive T cells.

148. SUBJECT AREA: The need for organized lymphoid tissue
QUESTION: Which of the following lymphoid tissues is unencapsulated:

> *A:* Thymus
> *B:* Lymph node
> *C:* Spleen
> *D:* Tonsil
> *E:* MALT

☐ Correct Answer: *E*

Learning Response A: Incorrect. The thymus is encapsulated by a layer of connective tissue.

Learning Response B: Incorrect. The lymph nodes are encapsulated by a layer of connective tissue.

Learning Response C: Incorrect. The spleen is encapsulated by a layer of connective tissue.

Learning Response D: Incorrect. The tonsils are encapsulated by a layer of connective tissue.

Learning Response E: Correct. The respiratory, alimentary and genitourinary tracts are guarded immunologically by subepithelial accumulations of lymphoid tissues which are not constrained by a connective tissue capsule. These may occur as diffuse collections of lymphocytes, plasma cells and phagocytes throughout the body and the lamina propria of the intestinal wall, or as more clearly organized tissue with well-formed follicles as found in the Peyer's patches.

149. SUBJECT AREA: Core revision
QUESTION: LFA-1 belongs to which family of molecules:

A: Complement receptors
B: Cytokine receptors
C: Integrins
D: VLA
E: MEL-14

☐ Correct Answer: *C*

Learning Response A: Incorrect. But a molecule which is closely related to LFA-1 is the CR3 complement receptor which binds C3bi and also shares the ligand ICAM-1 with the LFA-1 molecule.

Learning Response B: Incorrect. There are specific receptors for each cytokine, although some of them share one or more chains in common. However, LFA-1 does not function in any of the cytokine receptors.

Learning Response C: Correct. The integrin superfamily is, in general, concerned with tissue migration of cells during embryogenesis, tumor metastasis, wound healing, thrombosis and helper and cytotoxic T-cell functions. Some, such as LFA-1 which binds ICAM-1, mediate intercellular adhesion whilst others, such as the VLA molecules, are perhaps more concerned with adhesion to extracellular matrix components. They are heterodimers with unique but related α chains which can be grouped into subsets, each of which has a common β chain.

Learning Response D: Incorrect. The VLA molecules form a subset of the integrin family with a common β_1 chain distinct from the subset containing LFA-1. The VLA molecules take their name from VLA-1 and VLA-2 which appear as 'very late' antigens on T cells 2-4 weeks after in vitro activation. However, VLA-3, -4 and -5 are not 'very late' and are found to differing extents on lymphocytes, monocytes, platelets and probably hematopoietic progenitors.

Learning Response E: Incorrect. MEL-14 is a monoclonal antibody which recognizes the L-selectin lymphocyte homing receptor which binds to the vascular addressin on the surface of endothelial cells.

---

150. SUBJECT AREA: Lymphocytes traffic between lymphoid tissues
QUESTION: The VLA molecules are:

> *A:* Homotrimers
> *B:* Homodimers
> *C:* Single chain molecules
> *D:* Heterodimers with a common β chain
> *E:* Heterodimers with a common α chain

☐ Correct Answer: *D*

Learning Response A: Incorrect. These 'very late antigens' are members of the integrin family of adhesion molecules, but are not homotrimers.

Learning Response B: Incorrect. These 'very late antigens' are members of the integrin family of adhesion moleclues, but are not homodimers.

Learning Response C: Incorrect. These 'very late antigens' are members of the integrin family of adhesion moleclues, but are not single chain molecules.

Learning Response D: Correct. The α chain is specific for each VLA molecule (e.g. VLA-1 is an $\alpha_1\beta_1$ molecule, whereas VLA-6 is an $\alpha_6\beta_1$ molecule).

Learning Response E: Incorrect. They possess α chains but these are specific for each VLA molecule.

151. SUBJECT AREA: Encapsulated lymph nodes
QUESTION: On entering a germinal center, the primary B-blasts grow exponentially to form:

- *A:* Secondary B-blasts
- *B:* Centrocytes
- *C:* Centroblasts
- *D:* Memory B cells
- *E:* Plasma cells

☐ Correct Answer: *C*

Learning Response A: Incorrect. Secondary B-blasts are found in the apical light zone and are derived from centrocytes.

Learning Response B: Incorrect. Centrocytes are found in the basal light zone, are formed from centroblasts, are noncycling and begin to upregulate their expression of surface immunoglobulin. At this stage there is very extensive apoptotic cell death giving rise to DNA fragments which are visible as tingible bodies within the macrophages—the final resting place of the dead cells.

Learning Response C: Correct. Centroblasts are found in the dark zone and are highly mitotic cells with no surface IgD and very little surface IgM.

Learning Response D: Incorrect. Memory B cells are formed from secondary B cell blasts and either take up residence in the mantle zone or join the recirculating B-cell pool.

Learning Response E: Incorrect. Plasma cells are formed from the secondary B cell blasts and, being specialized for the secretion of large amounts of antibody, have a well-defined endoplasmic reticulum, prominent Golgi apparatus and cytoplasmic immunoglobulin. They migrate to the medullary cords which project between the medullary sinuses.

152. SUBJECT AREA: Encapsulated lymph nodes
QUESTION: In a lymph node, the antigen pneumococcus polysaccharide SIII leads to:

- *A:* Lymphocyte proliferation in the paracortex
- *B:* PALS development
- *C:* Development of cellular hypersensitivity

D: Proliferation in cortical lymphoid follicles
E: The absence of germinal centers

☐ Correct Answer: *D*

Learning Response A: Incorrect. Pneumococcus polysaccharide SIII is a thymus-independent antigen, so the paracortex, being mainly a T-cell area, is not significantly involved.

Learning Response B: Incorrect. The periarteriolar lymphoid sheath (PALS) is found in the spleen, not in the lymph node.

Learning Response C: Incorrect. Pneumococcus polysaccharide SIII is a thymus-independent antigen and therefore cellular (T cell) hypersensitivity does not ensue.

Learning Response D: Correct. Stimulation of antibody-formation by this thymus-independent antigen leads to proliferation in this location with development of germinal centers while the paracortical region remains inactive, reflecting the inability to develop cellular hypersensitivity to the polysaccharide.

Learning Response E: Incorrect. Germinal centers are produced during the response to both T-dependent and T-independent antigens.

153. SUBJECT AREA: Lymphocyte activation
QUESTION: CD8 is a marker of:

A: B cells
B: Helper T cells
C: Cytotoxic T cells
D: An activated macrophage
E: A polymorph precursor

☐ Correct Answer: *C*

Learning Response A: Incorrect. B cells bear surface marker CD19 and surface Ig receptor.

Learning Response B: Incorrect. Helper T cells bear CD4 as well as the CD3/T-cell receptor.

Learning Response C: Correct. CD8$^+$ T-cell receptor on the cytotoxic T cell, recognize the MHC class I + peptide on the target cell surface.

Learning Response D: Incorrect. Activated macrophages express increased class II, Fc receptors for IgG2b and binding sites for tumor cells.

Learning Response E: Incorrect.

---

154. SUBJECT AREA: Lymphocyte activation
QUESTION: CD4

   A: Is essentially an intracellular glycoprotein
   B: Is heterodimeric
   C: Binds processed peptide in its outer groove
   D: Binds to MHC class II on antigen-presenting cells
   E: Is highly polymorphic

☐ Correct Answer: D

Learning Response A: Incorrect. CD4 is a cell surface molecule.

Learning Response B: Incorrect. CD4 has a single peptide chain.

Learning Response C: Incorrect. The T-cell receptor binds processed peptide held in the outer groove of an MHC molecule.

Learning Response D: Correct. The CD4 binds to constant regions on the MHC class II.

Learning Response E: Incorrect.

---

155. SUBJECT AREA: Lymphocyte activation
QUESTION: The following is characteristic of B but not T cells:

   A: Class I MHC
   B: CD3
   C: Measles virus receptor
   D: Polyclonal activation of concanavalin A
   E: Surface immunoglobulin

☐ Correct Answer: *E*

Learning Response A: Incorrect. Class I MHC is present on both B and T cells.

Learning Response B: Incorrect. CD3 is present on T cells.

Learning Response C: Incorrect. This receptor is a feature of T cells.

Learning Response D: Incorrect. T cells but not B cells are polyclonally activated.

Learning Response E: Correct. B cells express the surface immunoglobulin of specificity created by that cell's particular immunoglobulin gene recombinations. A totally different gene set encodes the T-cell receptor for antigen.

---

156. SUBJECT AREA: Lymphocyte activation
QUESTION: A resting naive T cell engages its specific MHC/peptide complex displayed on the surface of a fibroblast. This leads to:

    A: Blast cell formation
    B: Induction of IL-2 production
    C: Activation of the T cell from G0 to G1
    D: Anergy
    E: Secretion of IL-1

☐ Correct Answer: *D*

Learning Response A: Incorrect. The naive T-cell receptor recognizes the MHC/peptide complex but in the absence of a costimulator such as B7 on the antigen-presenting cell, the T cell does not proliferate. An already activated T cell, however, would proliferate in the absence of the costimulator.

Learning Response B: Incorrect.

Learning Response C: Incorrect. In the absence of costimulator, the cell is not activated.

Learning Response D: Correct. In the absence of costimulator, a cell becomes anergic and incapable of subsequent response to the specific antigen.

Learning Response E: Incorrect.

157. SUBJECT AREA: Lymphocyte activation
QUESTION: The T-cell ligand binding B7 on a professional antigen-presenting cell is:

   A: CD28
   B: CD2
   C: LFA-1
   D: ICAM-1
   E: VCAM-1

☐ Correct Answer: *A*

Learning Response A: Correct. The ligand of precursor cytotoxic cells is CTLA-4.

Learning Response B: Incorrect. The ligand for CD2 is LFA-3.

Learning Response C: Incorrect. The ligand for LFA-1 is ICAM-1.

Learning Response D: Incorrect. The ligand for ICAM-1 is LFA-1.

Learning Response E: Incorrect. The ligand for VCAM-1 is VLA-4.

158. SUBJECT AREA: Lymphocyte activation
QUESTION: Proliferation of activated T cells:

   A: Is stimulated by a single signal induced by engagement of the T-cell receptor
   B: Requires both the signal described in A plus costimulation from B7 or p39
   C: Requires both the 2 signals described in B plus interaction between LFA-1 and ICAM-1
   D: Requires only mutual binding of LFA-3 and CD2 on the antigen-presenting cell and T cell, respectively
   E: Is unaffected by mitomycin C

☐ Correct Answer: *A*

Learning Response A: Correct. Unlike naive T cells, activated T cells only require a single signal induced by engagement of the T-cell receptor with MHC/peptide and involvement of CD4 or CD8 recognizing the constant part of the MHC.

Learning Response B: Incorrect. This is true for naive T cells.

Learning Response C: Incorrect. The interaction between LFA-1 and ICAM-1 greatly facilitates the impact of the single T-cell receptor signal by improving the mutual binding of antigen-presenting cell and T cell.

Learning Response D: Incorrect. The binding of LFA-3 to CD2 improves the links between the APC and T cell but proliferation also requires engagement of the T-cell receptor. Combination of monoclonals which are anti-CD2 can themselves initiate proliferation.

Learning Response E: Incorrect. Proliferation requires synthesis of new mRNA.

159. SUBJECT AREA: Lymphocyte activation
QUESTION: Protein tyrosine kinase activity following T-cell stimulation:

   A: Phosphorylates and thereby activates phospholipase cγ1
   B: Is an inherent property of the T-cell receptor α and β chains
   C: Is an inherent property of the consensus motifs in CD3 peptide chains
   D: Is unaffected by herbimycin A
   E: Is unrelated to phosphorylation of the CD3-associated ζ (zeta) chains

☐ Correct Answer: *A*

Learning Response A: Correct. The tyrosine kinase activates the phospholipase which accelerates the hydrolysis of phosphatidylinositol diphosphate to diacyl glycerol and inositol triphosphate.

Learning Response B: Incorrect. The T-cell receptor does not have kinase activity but the chains associate with kinase molecules.

Learning Response C: Incorrect. The consensus motifs in CD3 probably associate with kinase molecules.

Learning Response D: Incorrect. Tyrosine kinase enzymes are inhibited by herbimycin A.

Learning Response E: Incorrect. The zeta chains are very rapidly phosphorylated following T-cell stimulation.

160. SUBJECT AREA: Lymphocyte activation
QUESTION: T-cell mutants lacking CD45 cannot transduce signals received through the specific T-cell receptor because CD45:

A: Has protein tyrosine kinase activity
B: Directly phosphorylates CD4
C: Is a calcium ion channel
D: Removes phosphate group from a negative regulatory site on the lck kinase
E: Acts as a nuclear transcription factor

☐ Correct Answer: *D*

Learning Response A: Incorrect. CD45 has phosphatase rather than kinase activity.

Learning Response B: Incorrect. Molecule is a phosphatase.

Learning Response C: Incorrect. CD45 is not a calcium channel although on activation of T-cells these channels open.

Learning Response D: Correct. In the CD45 deficient cells, the lck is phosphorylated on tyrosine 505, a negative regulatory site for kinase activity.

Learning Response E: Incorrect. CD45 is a surface membrane molecule.

161. SUBJECT AREA: Lymphocyte activation
QUESTION: The early increase in phospholipase Cγ1 activity following T-cell stimulation:

A: Represents a sensitive regulatory negative feedback control mechanism
B: Dephosphorylates protein tyrosine kinase inhibitors
C: Accelerates hydrolysis of diacyl glycerol
D: Accelerates hydrolysis of phosphatidylinositol diphosphate
E: Accelerates hydroylsis of inositol triphosphate

☐ Correct Answer: *D*

Learning Response A: Incorrect. The phospholipase is part of the stimulatory mechanism.

Learning Response B: Incorrect. The enzyme splits phospholipids but it is not a phosphatase.

Learning Response C: Incorrect. The enzyme forms diacyl glycerol.

Learning Response D: Correct. The enzyme splits phosphatidylinositol diphosphate to diacyl glycerol and inositol triphosphate.

Learning Response E: Incorrect. The enzyme forms inositol triphosphate.

---

162. SUBJECT AREA: Lymphocyte activation
QUESTION: The nuclear AP-1 site responsible for 90% of IL-2 enhancer activity:

    A: Binds the Oct-1 transcriptional factor
    B: Binds proteins encoded by the Fos/Jun proto oncogenes
    C: Binds the nuclear factor of activated T cells (NFAT)
    D: Binds the NF-κB transcriptional factor
    E: Binds polyclonal mitogenic agents such as concanavalin A

☐ Correct Answer: *B*

Learning Response A: Incorrect. Oct-1 binds to the antigen receptor response element 1 (ARRE-1).

Learning Response B: Correct.

Learning Response C: Incorrect. NFAT binds to ARRE-2.

Learning Response D: Incorrect.

Learning Response E: Incorrect. Polyclonal mitogenic agents such as Con A bind to receptors on the cell surface.

---

163. SUBJECT AREA: B-lymphocyte activation
QUESTION: A lipopolysaccharide (LPS) from Gram-negative bacteria is:

A: A thymus-dependent antigen
B: A type 2 thymus-independent antigen
C: A polyclonal activator of murine B cells
D: Cross-links Ig receptors on B cells
E: Produces high affinity IgG memory responses

☐ Correct Answer: *C*

Learning Response A: Incorrect. LPS stimulates B cells without the presence of T cells.

Learning Response B: Incorrect. LPS stimulates T cells without reacting with the Ig receptors; type 2 thymus-independent antigens are polymeric and combine with and cross-link Ig receptors.

Learning Response C: Correct. LPS reacts with a specific receptor on most murine B cells and therefore is not selective for B cells of any particular antigen specificity.

Learning Response D: Incorrect. LPS does not react with Ig receptors except on the specific B cells that have surface Ig complementary to LPS itself.

Learning Response E: Incorrect. Since the response is thymus-independent, high affinity IgG memory responses cannot be produced.

164. SUBJECT AREA: B-lymphocyte activation
QUESTION: The carrier T-cell epitope on a thymus-dependent antigen:

A: Behaves like a hapten
B: Needs to be polymeric
C: Need not be physically connected to the B-cell epitope
D: Is a carbohydrate
E: Stimulates help for the B-cell response

☐ Correct Answer: *E*

Learning Response A: Incorrect. The antigen possessing the carrier epitope binds to the B cell but unlike a hapten, it will stimulate the T cell provided of course T cells are also present.

Learning Response B: Incorrect. It can be univalent unlike type 2 T-independent antigens which are polymeric and cross-link Ig receptors.

Learning Response C: Incorrect. It is essential for T- and B-cell epitopes to be connected because the B cell captures the antigen through the B-cell epitope, processes the antigen and presents the peptide from the T-cell epitope to the helper T cell.

Learning Response D: Incorrect. Carbohydrates are not processed to form T-cell epitopes.

Learning Response E: Correct. The presentation of the T-cell epitope by the B-cell recruits the T-cell help for activating the B cell causing its proliferation and final maturation.

---

165. SUBJECT AREA: B-lymphocyte activation
QUESTION: T-cell help for antibody production:

- *A:* Depends on T-cell recognition of native antigen bound to B-cell surface Ig
- *B:* Depends on T-cell recognition of antigen processed by the B cell
- *C:* Involves class I MHC on the B cell
- *D:* Can occur in X-irradiated mice
- *E:* Is a feature of the antibody response to pneumococcal polysaccharide SIII

☐ Correct Answer: *B*

Learning Response A: Incorrect. T cells do not recognize native antigen.

Learning Response B: Correct. The native antigen binds to B-cell surface Ig, is taken inside the cell, processed and the peptide placed as a complex with class II MHC on the cell surface where it is recognized by T-helper cells.

Learning Response C: Incorrect. Cytotoxic cells recognize class I MHC plus peptide whereas helper cells see class II.

Learning Response D: Incorrect. The clonal expansion required for effective antibody production cannot occur after X-irradiation which inhibits cell division.

Learning Response E: Incorrect. Pneumococcal polysaccharide cannot be processed for presentation with class II MHC and is therefore thymus-independent as an antigen.

166. SUBJECT AREA: B-lymphocyte activation
QUESTION: Cross-linking of B-cell surface receptors:

- A: Is a feature of thymus-dependent antigens
- B: Lowers the intracellular Ca^{++} concentration
- C: Rapidly phosphorylates the Ig-α and Ig-β chains of the surface Ig receptor
- D: Requires contiguity of 2 B-cell epitopes of different specificity on the same antigen molecule
- E: Cannot be achieved by anti-idiotypic antibodies

☐ Correct Answer: *C*

Learning Response A: Incorrect. Thymus-dependent antigens may be univalent and are processed after binding to the cell surface Ig.

Learning Response B: Incorrect. The intracellular calcium concentration is increased on activation.

Learning Response C: Correct. This results from very rapid activation of kinases. Of these, the B-cell–specific, blk src kinase, is activated within 1 minute.

Learning Response D: Incorrect. This cannot occur because all the surface receptors on a given B cell have the same specificity.

Learning Response E: Incorrect. Because they are bivalent, anti-Id can cross-link to surface receptors bearing idiotype.

167. SUBJECT AREA: B-lymphocyte activation
QUESTION: Activation of resting B cells by T-helpers depends directly upon costimulatory interaction between:

- A: CD40 and p39
- B: B7 and CD28
- C: B7 and CTLA-4
- D: CD4 and MHC class II
- E: ICAM-1 and LFA-1

☐ Correct Answer: *A*

Learning Response A: Correct.

Learning Response B: Incorrect. This interaction activates T-helper cells.

Learning Response C: Incorrect. This interaction activates cytotoxic cell precursors.

Learning Response D: Incorrect. This interaction in itself is one part of the recognition of antigen-presenting cells by T cells but without the CD40/p39 costimulatory interaction, resting cells cannot be activated.

Learning Response E: Incorrect. These molecules help the initial interaction between APC and T-helpers by increasing adhesiveness but probably do not contribute to signalling.

168. SUBJECT AREA: Core revision
QUESTION: B cells as distinct from T cells:

- *A:* Are polyclonally activated by phytohemagglutinin
- *B:* Bear surface Ig receptors for antigen
- *C:* Bear surface CD3 molecules
- *D:* Are activated by streptococcal exotoxin superantigens
- *E:* Have surface receptors for measles virus

☐ Correct Answer: *B*

Learning Response A: Incorrect. Phytohemagglutinin is a polyclonal activator of T-cells independently of their T-cell receptor specificity.

Learning Response B: Correct. The specific receptor for antigen on B cells is surface immunoglobulin whereas that on T cells is made up of the α- and β-chains.

Learning Response C: Incorrect. The T-cell receptor transduces its signal through the chains of the CD3 complex.

Learning Response D: Incorrect. These superantigens act by cross-linking MHC II with the $V\beta$ region of the T-cell surface receptor.

Learning Response E: Incorrect. Receptors for measles virus are present on T cells.

169. SUBJECT AREA: Core revision
QUESTION: The T-cell receptor link to MHC/peptide is enhanced by interaction between MHC class II on the antigen-presenting cells with the following molecule on the T cell:

   A: LFA-1
   B: CD2
   C: CD4
   D: CD8
   E: CD28

☐ Correct Answer: *C*

Learning Response A: Incorrect. LFA-1 binds to ICAM-1.

Learning Response B: Incorrect. CD2 binds to LFA-3.

Learning Response C: Correct. CD4 on helper T cells binds to the non-polymorphic part of the MHC class II molecule.

Learning Response D: Incorrect. CD8 on cytotoxic T cells binds to the non-polymorphic part of MHC class I on the antigen-presenting or target cell.

Learning Response E: Incorrect. CD28 is ligated by the B7 molecule on the antigen-presenting cell.

170. SUBJECT AREA: Core revision
QUESTION: The costimulatory signal for activation of resting T cells is provided by ligation of:

   A: CD28
   B: Surface Ig
   C: LFA-1
   D: VLA-4
   E: IL-2

☐ Correct Answer: *A*

Learning Response A: Correct. B7 on the antigen-presenting cell ligating with CD28 on the T cell provides a costimulatory signal for T-cell activation.

Learning Response B: Incorrect. B cells do not provide a costimulatory signal for resting T cells. However, surface Ig on B cells can pick up antigen which can then be processed and presented to activated T-helper cells.

Learning Response C: Incorrect. LFA-1, by binding to ICAM-1, augments activation signals but does not provide a costimulatory signal necessary for activation of resting T cells.

Learning Response D: Incorrect. VLA-4 which binds to VCAM-1 on the antigen-presenting cell does not provide a costimulatory signal but does augment the effect of other signals.

Learning Response E: Incorrect. The cytokine, IL-2, binding to the IL-2 receptor will cause proliferation of activated T cells.

171. SUBJECT AREA: Core revision
QUESTION: One of the earliest events in T-cell signalling is:

    A: Activation of phospholipase C
    B: Activation of protein kinase C
    C: Production of inositol triphosphate
    D: Activation of protein tyrosine kinase
    E: Mobilization of cellular calcium

☐ Correct Answer: *D*

Learning Response A: Incorrect. Phospholipase C is activated by phosphorylation and then splits phosphatidylinositol diphosphate.

Learning Response B: Incorrect. Protein kinase C becomes activated by diacyl glycerol produced through the action of phospholipase C.

Learning Response C: Incorrect. Inositol triphosphate is produced from phosphatidylinositol diphosphate by the action of phospholipase C.

Learning Response D: Correct. Activation of protein tyrosine kinase activity is responsible for subsequent activation of membrane components by phosphorylation.

Learning Response E: Incorrect. Intracellular calcium is mobilized at a later stage through binding of inositol triphosphate to specific receptors on specialized calcium storage vesicles.

172. SUBJECT AREA: Core revision

QUESTION: On injection into mice, bovine serum albumin conjugated with dinitrophenol (DNP) behaves as a:

A: Type 1 thymus-independent antigen
B: Type 2 thymus-independent antigen
C: Thymus-dependent antigen
D: Polyclonal T-cell activator
E: Hapten

☐ Correct Answer: *C*

Learning Response A: Incorrect. Type 1 thymus-independent antigens are polyclonal activators like LPS which bind to specific receptors on the lymphocyte, focused there by surface immunoglobulins specific for the polyclonal activator.

Learning Response B: Incorrect. Type 2 thymus-independent antigens are polymeric molecules which cross-link surface Ig.

Learning Response C: Correct. BSA-DNP is thymus-dependent in that the BSA acts as a T-dependent carrier which is processed by an anti-DNP B cell which binds the conjugate and presents the processed peptide with MHC to the T-helper cell. The T cell helps the B cell to mature into an anti-DNP clone.

Learning Response D: Incorrect. Examples of polyclonal T-cell activators are phytohemagglutinin and concanavalin A.

Learning Response E: Incorrect. The DNP is a hapten in that it will bind to preformed antibody, particularly on the surface of the B cell, but will not itself stimulate antibody formation until conjugated to a T-dependent carrier such as the bovine serum albumin.

173. SUBJECT AREA: Core revision

QUESTION: T cell p39 provides a costimulatory signal to B cells by ligating:

A: Surface Ig
B: MHC class II
C: CD28
D: CD19
E: CD40

☐ Correct Answer: *E*

Learning Response A: Incorrect. Surface Ig ligates specific antigen.

Learning Response B: Incorrect. MHC class II bearing processed peptide ligates the T-cell receptor and CD4/8.

Learning Response C: Incorrect. CD28 ligates the costimulatory molecule B7 on an antigen presenting cell.

Learning Response D: Incorrect. CD19 is a pan-B-cell surface molecule of unknown function.

Learning Response E: Correct. The co-stimulatory signal provided by the p39/CD40 interaction is necessary for the activation of resting B cells in addition to the TCR interaction.

174. SUBJECT AREA: Core revision
QUESTION: Cytokines:

    A: Are usually around 150-200 kDa
    B: Have glycosyl phosphatidylinositol (GPI) anchors
    C: Are pleiotropic
    D: Generally act at long range
    E: Produce very stable long-lived messenger RNA

☐ Correct Answer: *C*

Learning Response A: Incorrect. The basic 'monomeric' (four chain) immunoglobulin structure has a molecular mass in this range.

Learning Response B: Incorrect. Although some cytokines may be found on membranes, they are not thought to use transmembrane or GPI anchors.

Learning Response C: Correct. Cytokines can exhibit multiple effects on growth, differentiation and activation of a variety of cell types.

Learning Response D: Incorrect. Most cytokines act transiently and usually at short range, although circulating IL-1 and IL-6 can mediate release of acute phase proteins from the liver.

Learning Response E: Incorrect. AU-rich regions in the 3'-untranslated region of the mRNA for many cytokines are associated with rapid degradation of the mRNA and therefore cytokine production is short-lived in the absence of continued gene transcription.

---

175. SUBJECT AREA: Cytokines
QUESTION: Which set of cytokine genes are tightly linked on chromosome 5 in man:

  A: IL-3, IL-4, IL-5 and GM-CSF
  B: IL-1, IL-2, IL-3 and G-CSF
  C: TNFα and TNFβ
  D: VLA1-6
  E: G-CSF, M-CSF and GM-CSF

☐ Correct Answer: *A*

Learning Response A: Correct. Within the same region on chromosome 5 there are also genes for M-CSF and its receptor, and for several other growth factors and receptors.

Learning Response B: Incorrect. These cytokines are completely unlinked genetically, each being on a different chromosome (in man: IL-1 chromosome 2, IL-2 chromosome 4, IL-3 chromosome 5 and G-CSF on chromosome 17).

Learning Response C: Incorrect. TNFα and TNFβ are closely linked within the MHC class III region on chromosome 6 in man and chromosome 17 in mouse.

Learning Response D: Incorrect. VLA1-6 are heterodimeric molecules with a common β chain encoded on chromosome 10 in man, and individual α chains which are encoded on various chromosomes.

Learning Response E: Incorrect. G-CSF is on chromosome 17, whereas M-CSF and GM-CSF are within the same region on chromosome 5, although they are far enough apart to not be tightly linked.

---

176. SUBJECT AREA: Core revision
QUESTION: T_{h1} cells secrete:

  A: CD4
  B: IL-4
  C: IL-5

D: IL-10
E: Interferon-γ

☐ Correct Answer: *E*

Learning Response A: Incorrect. T_{h1} cells produce the CD4 molecule, as do T_{h2} cells, but this is a transmembrane-anchored cell surface molecule and is not actively secreted.

Learning Response B: Incorrect. Interleukin-4 is a typical T_{h2} cytokine which helps B cells to synthesize antibody. It is able to block both the proliferation of, and cytokine release by, T_{h1} cells.

Learning Response C: Incorrect. Interleukin-5 is a typical T_{h2} cytokine which helps B cells to synthesize antibody. IL-5 plus IL-4 promotes IgM synthesis, whereas IL-4, -5 and -6 (with a possible contribution from IFN-γ) stimulate IgG synthesis.

Learning Response D: Incorrect. Interleukin-10 is a typical T_{h2} cytokine and is able to block both proliferation and cytokine release by T_{h1} cells.

Learning Response E: Correct. T_{h1} cells are concerned with inflammatory processes, macrophage activation and delayed sensitivity. They produce IFNγ, IL-2, IL-3 and GM-CSF.

177. SUBJECT AREA: Cytokines
QUESTION: The αβ heterodimeric form of the IL-2 receptor:

A: Is downregulated on activated cells
B: Binds IL-2 with high affinity
C: Is found only on T cells
D: Uses CD45 as an α chain
E: Allows rapid dissociation of bound IL-2

☐ Correct Answer: *B*

Learning Response A: Incorrect. The αβ heterodimeric form of the IL-2 receptor is upregulated on activated cells.

Learning Response B: Correct. The αβ heterodimeric form of the IL-2 receptor has an affinity (K_a) of 10^{11} M^{-1}, whereas the α chain alone binds IL-2 with low affinity, and the β chain alone with medium affinity.

Learning Response C: Incorrect. Interleukin-2 was previously called T cell growth factor (TCGF), but the receptor is found not only on T cells but is also present on the surface of B cells and NK cells.

Learning Response D: Incorrect. The α chain of the IL-2 receptor is CD25, which reacts with the TAC monoclonal antibody. CD45 occurs in various isoforms and is a phosphatase sometimes referred to as the leukocyte common antigen.

Learning Response E: Incorrect. When the α and β chains form a single receptor, the α chain binds the IL-2 rapidly and facilitates its binding to a separate site on the β chain from which it can only dissociate slowly.

---

178. SUBJECT AREA: T-cell effectors in cell-mediated immunity
QUESTION: IFNγ and TNFβ can act synergistically because:

        A: TNFβ induces the formation of IFNγ receptors
        B: IFNγ prevents the formation of TNFβ receptors
        C: IFNγ induces the formation of TNFβ receptors
        D: They both bind to the same receptor
        E: They cross-link IFNγ and TNFβ receptors

☐ Correct Answer: *C*

Learning Response A: Incorrect. TNFβ can act in a cascade and induces the formation of IFNγ (and IL-1, GM-CSF and IL-6) but does not directly lead to the induction of the IFNγ receptor.

Learning Response B: Incorrect. IFNγ does show some antagonistic effects, e.g., antagonism of IL-4 and IFNγ on the transcription of silent mRNA preceding immunoglobulin class switching.

Learning Response C: Correct. IFNγ sets up the cell for destruction by inducing the formation of TNF receptors. Thus, there is synergism between IFNγ and TNFβ in the growth inhibition of the HeLa tumor cell line, and in the upregulation of surface MHC class II molecules on cultured pancreatic insulin-secreting cells.

Learning Response D: Incorrect. IFNγ and TNFβ bind to separate receptors.

Learning Response E: Incorrect. They bind to separate receptors and they do not bind to each other. Therefore they are unable to cross-link the IFNγ and TNFβ receptors.

179. SUBJECT AREA: Immunoglobulin class switching occurs in individual B cells
QUESTION: The cytokine which is most involved in the class switch to IgE production is:

  A: IL-1
  B: IL-2
  C: TGFβ
  D: IL-4
  E: IL-5

☐ Correct Answer: *D*

Learning Response A: Incorrect. IL-1 stimulates the proliferation of activated T and B cells, and induces prostaglandin E_2 (PGE_2) and cytokine production by macrophages.

Learning Response B: Incorrect. IL-2 stimulates the growth of activated T and B cells, and activates NK cells.

Learning Response C: Incorrect. TGFβ encourages cells to switch their immunoglobulin class to IgA, and IL-5 then stimulates them to become IgA secretors.

Learning Response D: Correct. Class switching to IgE can be induced by IL-4 alone, whereas IL-4 plus IL-5 tend to support IgM production and IL-4, -5, -6, probably together with IFNγ, are optimal for IgG production.

Learning Response E: Incorrect. IL-5 in combination with TGFβ stimulates IgA production, together with IL-4 stimulates IgM production, and together with IL-4, -6 and probably IFNγ stimulates IgG production.

180. SUBJECT AREA: Core revision
QUESTION: Which of the following is not a feature of germinal center B cells:

  A: Immunoglobulin gene class switching
  B: Apoptosis
  C: VDJ rearrangement
  D: Somatic hypermutation
  E: Proliferation

☐ Correct Answer: *C*

Learning Response A: Incorrect. Isotype switching occurs in the dark zone centroblasts.

Learning Response B: Incorrect. B-cell centroblasts die through apoptosis unless rescued by certain signals which upregulate *bcl-2*. These include cross-linking surface immunoglobulin by complexes on follicular dendritic cells, engagement of CD40 which drives the cell into the memory compartment, and soluble CD23 plus IL-1α which stimulates antibody formation.

Learning Response C: Correct. B cells entering the germinal center will have already rearranged their immunoglobulin genes.

Learning Response D: Incorrect. Somatic hypermutation in the dark zone centroblasts is followed by the selection of mutants by antigen which guides the development of high affinity B cells.

Learning Response E: Incorrect. There is clonal expansion (i.e., proliferation) occurring in the dark zone centroblasts.

181. SUBJECT AREA: The germinal center
QUESTION: In the germinal center, B cells are directed to become memory cells by:

A: CD40
B: CD23
C: IL-1α
D: IL-4
E: TGFβ

☐ Correct Answer: *A*

Learning Response A: Correct. Engagement of CD40 drives the cell to the memory compartment.

Learning Response B: Incorrect. CD23 is the low affinity IgE receptor, FcεRII, present on eosinophils, activated mature B cells and activated macrophages. Soluble CD23 stimulates the formation of plasma cells.

Learning Response C: Incorrect. IL-1α is a cytokine produced by macrophages and fibroblasts, which stimulates the proliferation of activated T and B cells, and induces prostaglandin E_2 (PGE_2) and cytokine production by macrophages. In the germinal center it stimulates the formation of plasma cells.

Learning Response D: Incorrect. IL-4 is a cytokine produced by $CD4^+$ T cells, mast cells and bone marrow stroma and which stimulates the proliferation of activated T and B cells, mast cells and hematopoietic precursors, induces MHC class II and FcεR expression on B cells, p75 IL-2R on T cells, isotype switch to IgG1 and IgE, and upregulation of macrophage antigen presentation and cytotoxic functions.

Learning Response E: Incorrect. TGFβ is produced by T and B cells and is involved in the isotype switch to IgA as well as having several inhibitory functions; such as inhibition of IL-2 receptor upregulation, IL-2 dependent lymphocyte proliferation, and IL-3 plus CSF-induced hematopoiesis.

182. SUBJECT AREA: Immunoglobulin class switching
QUESTION: The first event following the production of C_H sterile transcripts by immunoglobulin genes is:

A: VDJ rearrangement
B: Light chain rearrangement
C: Somatic hypermutation
D: Apoptosis
E: Class switching

☐ Correct Answer: *E*

Learning Response A: Incorrect. C_H sterile transcripts are not produced until after immunoglobulin V gene rearrangement has taken place. In immunoglobulin heavy chain loci, DJ rearrangement occurs first, followed by V to DJ rearrangement.

Learning Response B: Incorrect. C_H sterile transcripts are not produced until after immunoglobulin V gene rearrangement has taken place. In immunoglobulin light chain loci, this involves rearrangement of a V gene segment next to a J gene segment.

Learning Response C: Incorrect. Somatic hypermutation occurs both before and after the production of C_H sterile transcripts.

Learning Response D: Incorrect. Apoptosis occurs following either the failure to produce functional immunoglobulin gene rearrangements and therefore the inability to express immunoglobulin on the surface of the B cell, or following the delivery of an apoptotic signal if, for example, the receptor recognizes self antigen with high affinity.

Learning Response E: Correct. Sterile transcripts of a C_H gene, consisting of a 5' exon derived from the germ line sequence upstream of the relevent switch region, are associated with a switch to that class. Perhaps the transcripts facilitate the action of the recombinase in some way, or maybe they reflect an increased accessibility of that particular switch region to the enzyme.

183. SUBJECT AREA: Specificity of antibody
QUESTION: The specificity of antibody secreted by a B cell may not be the same as that of the surface Ig of the clonal parent because of:

- *A:* Class switching
- *B:* Somatic hypermutation
- *C:* Allelic exclusion
- *D:* Alternative splicing
- *E:* Different heavy–light pairing

☐ Correct Answer: *B*

Learning Response A: Incorrect. The term class switching refers to the utilization of different constant regions by the same VDJ rearranged gene sequence. Therefore, the process of class switching per se will not alter the antigen specificity of the antibody which is determined by the VDJ sequence.

Learning Response B: Correct. The specificity of antibody secreted by daughter cells is initially the same as that of the clonal parent, but later may deviate to some extent due to the high frequency of mutation as the clone expands.

Learning Response C: Incorrect. Allelic exclusion ensures that, in a given B cell, only the maternal or paternal allele is expressed, never both. This ensures that all the antibody produced by that B cell is of identical specificity.

Learning Response D: Incorrect. Alternative splicing is used by virgin B cells as a mechanism whereby both IgM and IgD can be co-expressed on the same cell. A primary RNA transcript is made which includes both $C\mu$ and $C\delta$ exons, and this is then processed to produce mRNA with either $C\mu$ or $C\delta$ sequences linked to the same VDJ rearranged sequence. The membrane and secreted forms of IgM are also obtained by alternative splicing.

Learning Response E: Incorrect. In a given B cell, due to allelic exclusion, only one allele (maternal or paternal) of the heavy chain, and only one allele of either the κ or λ light chain is expressed, and therefore the progeny will all have the same heavy:light pairing as the clonal parent. During ontogeny, there may be a switch to an alternative allele to escape from self-reactivity (receptor editing).

---

184. SUBJECT AREA: Core revision
QUESTION: Low amounts of antigen:

- A: Produce low affinity antibodies
- B: Do not influence the affinity of antibodies
- C: Produce high affinity antibodies
- D: Affect the avidity but not the affinity of antibodies
- E: Preferentially induce class switching

☐ Correct Answer: C

Learning Response A: Incorrect. Low amounts of antigen do not induce low affinity antibody. Note, however, that very low amounts of antigen can sometimes induce tolerance ('low zone tolerance') and that a point will be reached where antigen concentration is so low that it fails to elicit any kind of response.

Learning Response B: Incorrect. However, extremely low amounts of antigen may fail to be seen at all by the immune system.

Learning Response C: Correct. Low doses of antigen tend to select high affinity antibody since only these can be rescued in the germinal center. For the same reasons, affinity matures as antigen concentration falls during an immune response.

Learning Response D: Incorrect. The avidity (functional affinity) of the antibody is related to the affinity but also depends on the valency of antigen binding. The basic immunoglobulin 'monomer' (actually a tetramer of 2 heavy plus 2 light chains) has a valency of 2 because it possesses 2 antigen-binding arms. However, secretory IgA is a dimer with 4 antigen-binding arms and IgM a pentamer with 10 antigen-binding arms. IgM antibodies, although often of low intrinsic affinity, can be of high avidity.

Learning Response E: Incorrect. Class switching is under T-cell control, rather than being determined by the concentration of antigen.

---

185. SUBJECT AREA: Specificity of antibody
QUESTION: High affinity B-cell clones are usually generated by:

A: Somatic mutation
B: Expression of high affinity precursors in the virgin B-cell population
C: Class switching
D: Apoptosis
E: Gene conversion

☐ Correct Answer: A

Learning Response A: Correct. Class-switched B cells are subject to high mutation rates after the initial response. The normal V region mutation rate is of the order of 10^{-5}/base pair/cell division but this rises to 10^{-3} in B cells as a result of antigenic stimulation. Randomly, some of the mutated daughter cells will have higher affinity for antigen, some the same and some lower. B cells expressing antibody of increased affinity will be preferentially selected by antigen.

Learning Response B: Incorrect. The pre-immune B cell expresses IgM antibodies which frequently bear germ line V genes. These are generally of low affinity for antigen, although often 'polyreactive' in that they are able to bind, albeit weakly, to a number of different antigens.

Learning Response C: Incorrect. Class switching per se does not generate high affinity clones, although IgG and IgA antibodies are usually of higher affinity than IgM.

Learning Response D: Incorrect. Apoptosis is a form of programmed cell death characterized by nuclear degradation. Dead cells are clearly not a useful source of antibody of any affinity.

Learning Response E: Incorrect. Gene conversion will usually change a stretch of nucleotides in a gene and is therefore perhaps more likely to destroy the original antigen-binding specificity than increase the affinity for that antigen. Note, however, that avian species use gene conversion as a means of creating immunoglobulin diversity.

186. SUBJECT AREA: Core revision
QUESTION: Activated memory T cells can be defined on the basis of expression of:

A: T-cell receptor
B: Immunoglobulin
C: MHC class II molecules

D: CD45RO
E: CD45RA

☐ Correct Answer: *D*

Learning Response A: Incorrect. All T cells express a T-cell receptor, either the αβ or γδ heterodimer.

Learning Response B: Incorrect. T cells do not express immunoglobulin, which is a property restricted solely to B cells. When immunoglobulin is observed on the surface of T cells it is present by virtue of having bound to cell surface Fc receptors.

Learning Response C: Incorrect. In man, although not in the mouse, MHC class II gene products are expressed on the surface of activated T cells. This is not, however, a specific marker of memory T cells.

Learning Response D: Correct. CD45, the leukocyte common antigen, is found in various isoforms which are generated by alternative splicing. Activated memory and naive T cells are distinguished by expression of CD45 isoforms. Memory T cells have the CD45RO phenotype, whereas naive T cells are CD45RA$^+$. However, it seems likely that a proportion of the CD45RO population reverts to a CD45RA pool of *resting* memory cells, which rather confuses the issue with respect to memory but not activation.

Learning Response E: Incorrect. CD45, the leukocyte common antigen, is found in various isoforms which are generated by alternative splicing. CD45RA is largely a marker of naive T cells, although there is thought to be a pool of resting memory cells which are also CD45RA$^+$.

187. SUBJECT AREA: The synthesis of antibody
QUESTION: Prior to class switching, B cells express:

A: IgA alone
B: IgA and IgG
C: IgM and IgD
D: IgD alone
E: No surface Ig

☐ Correct Answer: *C*

Learning Response A: Incorrect. IgA is not found prior to class switching.

Learning Response B: Incorrect. B cells coexpressing IgA and IgG are not usually seen.

Learning Response C: Correct. Differential splicing allows coexpression of IgM and IgD with identical V regions on a single cell. IgD is lost upon antigen stimulation so that memory B cells lack this class of immunoglobulin.

Learning Response D: Incorrect. IgD is not expressed alone on the surface of any type of B-cell, but rather is always found in combination with IgM and sometimes additionally with either IgA or IgG.

Learning Response E: Incorrect. As B cells, by definition, express surface immunoglobulin this cannot be the right answer. Note, however, that pre-B cells lack surface immunoglobulin but possess intracytoplasmic μ heavy chain, and also that plasma cells progressively lose their surface Ig.

---

188. SUBJECT AREA: Genes upregulated by T-cell activation
QUESTION: Which is the first of the following genes to be upregulated subsequent to T-cell activation:

    A: CD23
    B: Cytokine receptor
    C: Cytokine
    D: Transcription factors concerned with G0 to G1 progression
    E: Adhesion molecules

☐ Correct Answer: *D*

Learning Response A: Incorrect. CD23 is the low affinity FcεRII which is found on activated mature B cells, activated macrophages, and on eosinophils.

Learning Response B: Incorrect. Cytokine receptor expression occurs up to 14 hours following stimulation.

Learning Response C: Incorrect. Cytokine expression occurs up to 14 hours following stimulation.

Learning Response D: Correct. Within 15–30 minutes these genes, including *c-myc* together with transcription factors involved in the control of IL-2 expression such as NF-AT, are expressed. A complex series of tyrosine and serine/threonine phosphorylation reactions produce the factors which push the cell into the mitotic cycle and drive clonal proliferation.

Learning Response E: Incorrect. The expression of the genes encoding adhesion molecules may occur only several days after the initial activation stimulus, for example, 7–14 days for the 'very late antigen' VLA-1, a member of the integrin superfamily involved in adhesion to extracellular matrix proteins.

---

189. SUBJECT AREA: Core revision
QUESTION: Which one of the following cytokines can mediate release of acute phase proteins from the liver:

- *A:* IL-10
- *B:* TGFβ
- *C:* IL-6
- *D:* IL-12
- *E:* LIF

☐ Correct Answer: *C*

Learning Response A: Incorrect. IL-10 is produced by Th2 cells, inhibits IFNγ secretion, and is generally an inhibitory cytokine which downregulates inflammatory processes.

Learning Response B: Incorrect. Generally acting as an inhibitory cytokine, transforming growth factor β is produced by both T and B lymphocytes and as well as promoting wound repair and angiogenesis it is able to cause neoplastic transformation of some normal cells. Immunoregulatory properties include inhibition of IL-2 receptor upregulation and of IL-2 dependent T- and B-cell proliferation. It also mediates the isotype switch to IgA.

Learning Response C: Correct. IL-6, like IL-1, can mediate release of acute phase proteins from the liver which suggests that, unlike most cytokines, they do not function only as short range mediators.

Learning Response D: Incorrect. IL-12 is produced by T cells and is an important activator of NK cells.

Learning Response E: Incorrect. Leukemia inhibitory factor is produced by T cells and is able to induce the proliferation of embryonic stem cells without affecting their differentiation, and is also involved in the chemoattraction and activation of eosinophils.

190. SUBJECT AREA: Cytokines
  QUESTION: Which of the following is most commonly used for the assay of specific cytokines:

  A: Plaque-forming cell assay
  B: Immunoassay
  C: Immunoprecipitation
  D: Immunofluorescence
  E: Fluorescence quench

☐ Correct Answer: B

Learning Response A: Incorrect. The plaque-forming cell assay provides a means by which antibody secretion from individual B cells can be analyzed.

Learning Response B: Correct. Cytokines are commonly measured using cellular assay systems, e.g., the proliferative response of IL-2 dependent T-cell lines. However, the growing awareness of the pleiotropic and network effects of cytokines has alerted researchers to the possible pitfalls in many cytokine-dependent cell line systems. This has led to their increasing replacement by immunoassay kits which are also much quicker and simpler than the cellular assays, although they only measure the presence of a cytokine rather than its effect in a particular system.

Learning Response C: Incorrect. Immunoprecipitation relies on the detection of antigens by cross-linking with specific antibody. This is not generally used to detect cytokines, particularly given their low abundance and to some extent their relatively small molecular weight (usually <25kDa).

Learning Response D: Incorrect. Although cytokines produced within cells can be measured using intracytoplasmic fluorescence, these techniques are not as widely used as immunoassay of secreted cytokines.

Learning Response E: Incorrect. Fluorescence quench is a method used for measuring affinity, and is particularly appropriate for antibodies directed towards small haptens.

191. SUBJECT AREA: Cytokines
  QUESTION: Cytokines always act:

  A: By binding to specific receptors
  B: In an autocrine fashion

C: At long range
D: Antagonistically with other cytokines
E: Synergistically with other cytokines

☐ Correct Answer: *A*

Learning Response A: Correct. The cell-type specificity of cytokines is provided by the regulated expression of specific cytokine receptor genes. Many cytokine receptors consist of more than one polypeptide. For example, the IL-2 receptor is composed of an α chain (CD25, TAC) of low affinity and a β chain of intermediate affinity; when both are expressed together they form the high affinity IL-2 receptor.

Learning Response B: Incorrect. Although several cytokines (e.g., IL-2, IL-6) can act in an autocrine manner stimulating the same cell as that which produced it, this is not always the case as the cells may often not be simultaneously expressing the specific receptor for that cytokine. Cytokines are usually able to act in a paracrine fashion, stimulating other cells in the local environment.

Learning Response C: Incorrect. Although a few cytokines such as IL-6 can act systemically, most of them are short range mediators.

Learning Response D: Incorrect. However, they can sometimes act antagonistically, e.g., IL-4 and IFNγ act antagonistically on the transcriptional regulation of Ig class switch-associated sterile transcripts.

Learning Response E: Incorrect. However, they can sometimes act synergistically, e.g., TNF and IFNγ act synergistically in the upregulation of surface MHC class II expression on, for example, cultured pancreatic insulin-secreting cells.

---

192. SUBJECT AREA: Core revision
QUESTION: Memory T cells are:

A: Continuously produced directly from naive progenitors without the need for antigenic stimulation
B: Sustained by recurrent stimulation with antigen
C: Only present in primary immune responses
D: Switch from an $\alpha\beta$ to a $\gamma\delta$ T-cell receptor
E: Express germ line Ig V genes

☐ Correct Answer: *B*

Learning Response A: Incorrect. Preexisting receptors of relatively high affinity in the population of naive cells proliferate selectively through preferential binding to antigen and a proportion of these, expressing increased levels of accessory adhesion molecules (CD2, LFA-1, LFA-3, and ICAM-1) constitute the memory population.

Learning Response B: Correct. Most memory cells are subject to repeated stimulation from antigen and this makes it likely that most of the features associated with the CD45RO subset are in fact manifestations of activated cells.

Learning Response C: Incorrect. Memory cells of both the T- and B-cell lineages are generated during a primary immune reponse (in the case of the latter only with thymus-dependent antigens) and form the basis of the secondary immune response.

Learning Response D: Incorrect. T cells do not switch from one type of T-cell receptor to the other form. Memory T cells of the $\alpha\beta$ lineage are fairly well characterized but little is known about $\gamma\delta$ memory T cells.

Learning Response E: Incorrect. Memory T cells express T-cell receptor V genes, not immunoglobulin V genes which encode the antigen receptors found on B lymphocytes. However, the TCR V genes, unlike Ig V genes, do not undergo somatic hypermutation following antigen stimulation.

193. SUBJECT AREA: Memory cells
QUESTION: The major long term source of a foreign antigen in the body is:

- *A:* Anti-idiotype
- *B:* Complexes on the surface of follicular dendritic cells
- *C:* Antigen bound to the surface of B cells
- *D:* Antigenic peptides in the groove of MHC molecules
- *E:* There are no long term sources of foreign antigen in the body

☐ Correct Answer: *B*

Learning Response A: Incorrect. Although internal image anti-idiotypes can provide a conformational mimic of external antigen, this is not foreign antigen.

Learning Response B: Correct. Activated B-memory cells are sustained by recurrent stimulation with antigen present as long term immune complexes on the surface of follicular dendritic cells in the germinal centers.

Learning Response C: Incorrect. Antigen bound to the surface of B cells is usually quickly internalized and may then be processed for presentation to T cells.

Learning Response D: Incorrect. Antigenic peptides in the groove of MHC molecules are derived from processed foreign (and self) antigens. There is thought to be a continuous turnover of MHC-peptide complexes and thus this does not constitute a major long term source of antigen.

Learning Response E: Incorrect. Immunological memory, the basis of the acquired immune response, is dependent upon the continued presence of antigen which sustains activated memory cells by recurrent stimulation.

194.
SUBJECT AREA: Control of immune responses
QUESTION: A major factor regulating the adaptive immune response is:

- *A:* The neutrophil granulocyte
- *B:* Complement membrane attack complex
- *C:* C-reactive protein
- *D:* Antigen concentration
- *E:* Haptoglobin

☐ Correct Answer: *D*

Learning Response A: Incorrect. A granulocyte is a phagocytic cell which will take up and kill microorganisms coated with antibody and complement. The granulocyte is not an antigen-presenting cell.

Learning Response B: Incorrect. The membrane attack complex is inserted in cells at the final stages of complement activation, and leads to death of the cell.

Learning Response C: Incorrect. C-reactive protein, like the other acute phase proteins, is a general innate immune response to infection and is produced through stimulation of the liver by IL-1 or IL-6.

Learning Response D: Correct. Lymphocytes are directly driven by antigen. The concentration of antigen is important because the binding to the surface of responding B cells is necessary for continued stimulation. As the antigen concentration falls through catabolism or neutralization or complex formation with antibody, so the immune response diminishes. In this way the immune response is not maintained at a high level when the antigen has been eliminated.

Learning response *E:* Incorrect. The haptoglobin is a molecule which is present in plasma and binds free hemoglobin.

---

195. SUBJECT AREA: Antigenic competition
QUESTION: Antigenic competition:

- *A:* Involves competition between T-cell epitopes for the MHC groove
- *B:* Involves competition for available antibodies
- *C:* Is unrelated to the concept of dominant and subdominant epitopes
- *D:* Can only occur with cryptic epitopes
- *E:* Refers to the differential immunogenicity of the carbohydrate and protein moieties in a glycoprotein

☐ Correct Answer: *A*

Learning Response A: Correct. If a given epitopic peptide is produced by processing of the protein antigen in relatively high amounts and binds strongly to the MHC groove, it will compete favorably with peptides that appear in lower concentration and with lower binding affinity. Thus we have the hierarchy of dominant and subdominant epitopes with cryptic epitopes at such low concentration, they cannot usually be perceived by resting T cells.

Learning Response B: Incorrect. However, B cells directed to a given epitope which have expanded greatly may dominate the competition for antigen over B cells specific for a different epitope that are in a minority.

Learning Response C: Incorrect. Dominant epitopes are so named because they compete effectively with subdominant and cryptic epitopes.

Learning Response D: Incorrect. Cryptic epitopes are so named because they produce such a low abundance of MHC/peptide complex, that they do not initiate T-cell responses.

Learning Response E: Incorrect. Antigenic competition generally refers to epitope competition rather than competition between chemically different epitopes. However, the answer to B does introduce a concept whereby different epitopes can be competed for by different pools of expanded B-cell clones.

---

196. SUBJECT AREA: Antibody feedback control
QUESTION: Negative feedback on adaptive B-cell responses is mediated by:

A: Antigen specific IgM
B: Antigen specific IgG
C: Just antigen neutralization
D: Fcγ receptors on macrophages
E: F(ab')$_2$ anti-μ

☐ Correct Answer: *B*

Learning Response A: Incorrect. Antigen-specific IgM enhances the B-cell response and as this class appears early after exposure to antigen, this accelerates the first protective antibody response.

Learning Response B: Correct. Antigen-specific IgG complexes the antigen which then cross-links surface receptors on the B cell both for antigen and for the Fc region of IgG. As IgG antibodies appear later in the response, they do not inhibit antibody synthesis until substantial responses have been achieved. This negative feedback mechanism is the basis for anti-rhesus D prophylaxis, the prevention of hemolytic disease of the newborn due to rhesus incompatibility.

Learning Response C: Incorrect. F(ab')$_2$ can neutralize antigen but is far less effective at feedback control. Hence the word "just" in the question.

Learning Response D: Incorrect. B-cell Fcγ receptors are involved. Engagement of the macrophage Fcγ receptors leads to phagocytosis of IgG/Ag complexes.

Learning Response E: Incorrect. This reagent stimulates B-cell proliferation by acting as a type 2 thymus-independent antigen, cross-linking the surface IgM receptors on the B cell without engaging the inhibitory surface receptor for IgG.

197.
SUBJECT AREA: T-cell regulation
QUESTION: Injection of a mouse with a very high dose of sheep erythrocytes:

A: Induces a generalized antigen non-specific suppression
B: Induces antigen-specific T suppression
C: Depletes CD4 T cells
D: Increases CD8 T cells
E: Induces a high antibody response

☐ Correct Answer: *B*

Learning Response A: Incorrect. Suppression is antigen-specific.

Learning Response B: Correct. The suppression can be transferred by T cells and is specific for the antibody response to that antigen.

Learning Response C: Incorrect.

Learning Response D: Incorrect. There is no evidence for any significant increase in the numbers of CD8 T cells although conceivably there might be some proliferation of antigen-specific CD8 suppressor cells.

Learning Response E: Incorrect. The opposite is true.

198. SUBJECT AREA: T-cell regulation
QUESTION: Addition of anti-HLA-DQ to some lepromatous leprosy patients increases the proliferative response of their lymphocytes to *Mycobacterium leprae* suggesting:

    A: Cross-linking of T cells to antigen-presenting cells
    B: Increased processing of mycobacterial antigen
    C: Stimulation of activated T cells by anti-DQ
    D: Inhibition of antigen-specific T suppressors
    E: Stimulation by immune complexes

☐ Correct Answer: *D*

Learning Response A: Incorrect. If true, it would result in all DQ responsive T cells to the antigen showing increased proliferation.

Learning Response B: Incorrect. There is no mechanism for this to happen and if true, should occur with all antigen responsive DQ-restricted lymphocyte responses.

Learning Response C: Incorrect. There is no evidence for this. It should not occur with only certain patients if true. Also the effect is complement-dependent.

Learning Response D: Correct. The cells that respond are CD4 positive.

Learning Response E: Incorrect. The immune complexes would be those involving HLA-DQ and therefore should not be specific to *M. leprae*.

199.
SUBJECT AREA: T-cell regulation
QUESTION: Lepromin-specific CD8 suppressor clones established from lepromatous leprosy patients:

- A: Suppress EB virus transformed lepromin-specific B-cell lines
- B: Suppress lepromin-specific CD4 T cells in presence of antigen
- C: Lack T-cell receptors
- D: Are MHC-class I restricted
- E: Produce Th_1 type cytokines

☐ Correct Answer: *B*

Learning Response A: Incorrect. T-suppressors usually do not appear to have a direct effect on B cells.

Learning Response B: Correct. Proliferation is blocked.

Learning Response C: Incorrect.

Learning Response D: Incorrect. Surprisingly they are class II restricted unlike CD8 cytotoxic T cells.

Learning Response E: Incorrect. They produce Th_2-type cytokines which block Th_1 responses.

200.
SUBJECT AREA: T-cell regulation
QUESTION: Suppression of T_{h2} by T_{h1} cells may be mediated by:

- A: IL-2
- B: IL-3
- C: IL-4
- D: GM-CSF
- E: Interferon-γ

☐ Correct Answer: *E*

Learning Response A: Incorrect. IL-2 induces proliferation not suppression of Th_2 cells.

Learning Response B: Incorrect. Both Th$_1$ and Th$_2$ produce IL-3 and there is no evidence that it is suppressive to T cells.

Learning Response C: Incorrect. IL-4 is made Th$_2$ not Th$_1$ cells.

Learning Response D: Incorrect. Like IL-3, GM-CSF is made by both subtypes of helper cell.

Learning Response E: Correct.

201. SUBJECT AREA: T-cell regulation
QUESTION: Cells bearing MHC class I plus peptide are targets for specific:

A: B cells
B: Cytotoxic T cells
C: Th$_1$ cells
D: Th$_2$ cells
E: Interdigitating dendritic cells

☐ Correct Answer: *B*

Learning Response A: Incorrect. B cells have no receptors for MHC plus peptide.

Learning Response B: Correct. Cytotoxic T cells are guided by their antigen receptor plus CD8 to target cells bearing MHC class I plus peptide.

Learning Response C: Incorrect. Th$_1$ cells recognize MHC class II.

Learning Response D: Incorrect. Th$_2$ cells recognize MHC class II.

Learning Response E: Incorrect. Interdigitating dendritic cells are antigen-presenting cells and do not have receptors for MHC plus peptide.

202. SUBJECT AREA: Idiotype networks
QUESTION: Natural antibodies:

A: Are mostly IgG
B: Are mostly high affinity autoantibodies
C: Are produced spontaneously by CD5$^+$ B cells
D: Are acquired by transplacental passage from the mother
E: Do not arise in thymectomized mice

☐ Correct Answer: *C*

Learning Response A: Incorrect. They are essentially IgM.

Learning Response B: Incorrect. Although many are cross-reacting autoantibodies, they are of low affinity.

Learning Response C: Correct. They are produced by murine $CD5^+$ B cells without external antigenic stimulation.

Learning Response D: Incorrect. Since they are IgM, they do not cross the placenta.

Learning Response E: Incorrect. They are thymus-independent.

---

203. SUBJECT AREA: Idiotype networks
QUESTION: Monoclonal antibodies produced by hybridomas established from a single fetal mouse spleen frequently show mutual interaction. This is evidence for:

A: 'Sticky' neonatal Ig
B: Non-specific parallel sets
C: 'Private' idiotypes
D: Ig constant region interactions
E: An idiotype network present early in ontogeny of the immune system

☐ Correct Answer: *E*

Learning Response A: Incorrect. They do show antigen specificity although many of the neonatal antibodies are autoreactive and sometimes show wide cross-reactivity with several antigens.

Learning Response B: Incorrect. The non-specific parallel set represents a set of anti-idiotypes which have a common public idiotype ($Ab_{2\alpha}$).

Learning Response C: Incorrect. Private idiotypes represent idiotypic determinants present on one or a very restricted number of antibodies.

Learning Response D: Incorrect. The interactions are seen with $F(ab')_2$ fragments.

Learning Response E: Correct. Mutual interactions are idiotype–anti-idiotype. This frequency of mutual interaction is not seen if spleens are taken from adult mice.

---

204. SUBJECT AREA: Idiotype networks
QUESTION: The Jerne non-specific parallel idiotype set refers to:

- *A:* The idiotopes which make up an idiotype
- *B:* Antibodies of different specificity bearing the same idiotype
- *C:* The set of interacting idiotypes and anti-idiotypes
- *D:* Similar idiotypes in different strains of animal
- *E:* Parallel idiotypes on B and T cells

☐ Correct Answer: *B*

Learning Response A: Incorrect. An idiotope is an epitope on the antibody combining region which is recognized by a monoclonal antibody. Several of such antibodies found within an antiserum made against the original immunoglobulin, constitute an anti-idiotype serum.

Learning Response B: Correct. An idiotype which occurs fairly commonly on several different Ig species (public or cross-reactive idiotype) may often appear with increased frequency within the anti-idiotype antibodies which arise during an immune response.

Learning Response C: Incorrect. This refers to a whole network.

Learning Response D: Incorrect. These may be referred to as public or cross-reactive or common idiotypes, largely genetically controlled.

Learning Response E: Incorrect. However there are idiotypic connections between B and T cells.

---

205. SUBJECT AREA: Idiotype networks
QUESTION: Antibodies specific for different epitopes on the same antigen:

- *A:* Will bind to each other through idiotypic interactions
- *B:* Cannot bear similar idiotypes
- *C:* Can bear similar idiotypes independently of their antigenic specificity

D: Can only bear similar idiotypes if the antigenic epitopes cross-react

E: Must be of the same immunoglobulin class

☐ Correct Answer: *C*

Learning Response A: Incorrect. There is no reason for them to react with each other through idiotypes.

Learning Response B: Incorrect.

Learning Response C: Correct. Presumably an idiotype on an antibody to one epitope can induce either T-helper or immunoglobulin anti-idiotypes, which will selectively stimulate B cells directed to other epitopes on the same antigen which have a cross-reacting idiotype. Similarly, antibodies with a different specificity may also be stimulated and this will give rise to non-specific parallel sets.

Learning Response D: Incorrect. The phenomenon can work when the epitopes are completely unrelated. What is required are B cells which have been activated already by the response to the given antigen.

Learning Response E: Incorrect. Immunoglobulin class is related to heavy chain constant region which is not involved in idiotypic interactions.

206. SUBJECT AREA: Idiotype networks
QUESTION: Regulatory idiotypes on antibodies:

A: Are not usually 'public' idiotypes
B: Are not usually 'cross-reactive' idiotypes
C: Are usually common to several different antibodies
D: Are usually 'private' idiotypes
E: Are usually restricted to members of a single clone of antibodies

☐ Correct Answer: *C*

Learning Response A: Incorrect. Public idiotypes are present on the variable regions of a number of different antibodies. Regulation via idiotype can only have a significant affect on the overall immune response if the idiotype is fairly frequent, i.e., public.

Learning Response B: Incorrect. The term 'cross-reactive' idiotype is an alternative for 'public.'

Learning Response C: Correct. Regulation via idiotype can only have a significant affect on the overall immune response if the idiotype is fairly frequent, i.e. public, and the idiotype is common to a reasonable proportion of the antibodies making up the response. Public and cross-reactive are terms used to describe idiotypes common to several different antibodies.

Learning Response D: Incorrect. Private idiotypes are essentially restricted to a given immunoglobulin and would not qualify for a regulatory idiotype.

Learning Response E: Incorrect. Idiotype restricted to a single clone could not function widely as a regulatory idiotype.

207. SUBJECT AREA: Idiotype network
QUESTION: Anti-idiotypic immunoglobulins:

  A: Always suppress immune responses
  B: Can stimulate immune responses
  C: Can resemble their idiotype
  D: Cannot resemble the original antigen
  E: Are always IgM

☐ Correct Answer: *B*

Learning Response A: Incorrect. Suppression or stimulation through the idiotype may occur depending to some extent on the concentration of anti-Id injected. Stimulation and suppression may be seen during the course of immune responses *in vivo*, although the circumstances are not always fully understood.

Learning Response B: Correct. Suppression or stimulation through the idiotype may occur depending to some extent on the concentration of anti-Id injected. Stimulation and suppression may be seen during the course of immune responses *in vivo*, although the circumstances are not always fully understood.

Learning Response C: Incorrect. The anti-Id reacts with the idiotype and does not resemble it.

Learning Response D: Incorrect. A subset of anti-idiotypes which does resemble the original antigen is termed 'the internal image.'

Learning Response E: Incorrect. Anti-idiotypes are often IgG.

208. SUBJECT AREA: Idiotype network
QUESTION: An internal image monoclonal anti-idiotype:

- *A:* Has specificity for its own internal structure
- *B:* Is the mirror image of the idiotype
- *C:* Has identical idiotypes on heavy and light chains
- *D:* Mimics a single epitope on the antigen
- *E:* Cannot function as a 'surrogate' antigen

☐ Correct Answer: *D*

Learning Response A: Incorrect. The anti-idiotype will not react with itself.

Learning Response B: Incorrect. It reacts with and is complementary to the shape of the idiotype and will not be a mirror image.

Learning Response C: Incorrect. Idiotypes can be present on either heavy or light chains or more often on the combination. Identical structures giving identical anti-idiotypes on heavy and light chains would be very unlikely.

Learning Response D: Correct. It mimics a single epitope on the antigen because it derives from a paratope on the idiotype which reacts with a single epitope.

Learning Response E: Incorrect. It can react with antibodies to the original antigen and can provoke immune responses directed to the original antigen.

209. SUBJECT AREA: Genetic factors
QUESTION: High responder 'Biozzi' mice:

- *A:* Phagocytose carbon particles faster than low responders
- *B:* Kill intracellular bacteria more effectively than low responders
- *C:* Differ from low responders by a single gene
- *D:* Produce high titer antibodies to a restricted number of antigens
- *E:* Produce high titer antibodies to a variety of antigens

☐ Correct Answer: *E*

Learning Response A: Incorrect. High and low responders are equally effective at phagocytosis.

Learning Response B: Incorrect. The reverse is true. But high-responder macrophages present antigen more efficiently than low-responder macrophages, and are better at killing intracellular bacterial infections.

Learning Response C: Incorrect. More than 10 genes are involved in the differences.

Learning Response D: Incorrect. The ability to produce high titer antibodies extends over a fairly wide range of antigens since they were selected by response to the very complex series of antigens present on the red cell.

Learning Response E: Correct. The ability to produce high titer antibodies extends over a fairly wide range of antigens since they were selected by response to the very complex series of antigens present on the red cell.

210. SUBJECT AREA: Genetic factors
QUESTION: A high antibody response to an antigen such as (TG)-A-L in a given mouse strain:

- A: Is linked to immunoglobulin gene polymorphism
- B: Is independent of MHC (H-2) haplotype
- C: Depends on T-cell recognition of the antigen bound to MHC class II
- D: Depends on T-cell recognition of the antigen bound to MHC class I
- E: Reflects a general propensity to make high titer antibody responses

☐ Correct Answer: C

Learning Response A: Incorrect. Absence of an immunoglobulin variable gene may cause defective immune response to certain carbohydrate antigens such as dextran.

Learning Response B: Incorrect. It is dependent on the MHC haplotype. Alleles at the MHC will determine whether the given strain is a high or a low responder.

Learning Response C: Correct. If T cells recognize a fairly high concentration of MHC class II/processed peptide complex, there will be a good response. This will help the B cell to make antibody.

Learning Response D: Incorrect. The helper T cells need to recognize MHC class II. Cytotoxic cells recognize MHC class I/peptide.

Learning Response E: Incorrect. Strains giving a high response to TGAL may be poor responders to a different peptide such as HGAL. The general propensity for high antibody responses is a feature of Biozzi mice.

211. SUBJECT AREA: Genetic factors
QUESTION: Which of the following is never related to poor MHC-linked immune response:

   A: Defective T cell repertoire
   B: T-suppression
   C: Inadequate antigen processing
   D: Poor binding of peptide epitope to MHC
   E: Defective V gene rearrangement

☐ Correct Answer: *E*

Learning Response A: Incorrect. Cross-reaction between MHC derived epitope and a foreign epitope can lead to thymic depletion or tolerance so creating a hole in the repertoire.

Learning Response B: Incorrect. Dominant low responses in class II heterozygotes can indicate T-suppression.

Learning Response C: Incorrect. Certain individuals do not produce adequate concentrations of processed antigen peptide epitopes which fit with their MHC groove.

Learning Response D: Incorrect. Another way of stating that certain individuals do not produce adequate concentrations of processed antigen peptide epitopes which fit with their MHC groove.

Learning Response E: Correct. Rearrangements in the VDJ segments of the T-cell receptor are not related to the MHC genotype.

212. SUBJECT AREA: Neuroendocrine factors
QUESTION: Relative to males, females:

   A: Are less resistant to T-cell tolerance
   B: Are more susceptible to autoimmune disease
   C: Produce lower antibody responses to T-independent antigens

D: Have lower serum Ig levels
E: Have lower levels of secretory IgA

☐ Correct Answer: *B*

Learning Response A: Incorrect.

Learning Response B: Correct. Estrogenic oral contraceptives can exacerbate an autoimmune disease such as SLE. Male hormones can prolong the lifespan of NZBxW F1 females (murine model of SLE).

Learning Response C: Incorrect.

Learning Response D: Incorrect.

Learning Response E: Incorrect.

213. SUBJECT AREA: Influence of neuroendocrine factors
QUESTION: Immune responses are:

A: Depressed by stress
B: Stimulated by glucocorticoids
C: Depressed by estrogens
D: Stimulated by androgens
E: Depressed by growth hormone

☐ Correct Answer: *A*

Learning Response A: Correct. Stress induces glucocorticoids which are inhibitory.

Learning Response B: Incorrect. Glucocorticoids inhibit a variety of components of immune responses including inflammation.

Learning Response C: Incorrect. Estrogens tend to stimulate immune responses, particularly autoimmune phenomena.

Learning Response D: Inconrent. Androgens behave in the opposite way to estrogens which tend to stimulate immune responses, particularly autoimmune phenomena.

Learning Response E: Incorrect.

214. SUBJECT AREA: Influence of neuroendocrine factors
QUESTION: Stimulation of glucocorticoid synthesis by IL-1:

- *A:* Provides a basis for a feedback suppressor circuit
- *B:* Cannot provide a basis for a feedback suppressor circuit
- *C:* Augments IL-1 synthesis
- *D:* Augments cell-mediated immunity
- *E:* Augments IFNγ synthesis

☐ Correct Answer: *A*

Learning Response A: Correct. Glucocorticoids can act as a negative feedback because they suppress immune responses and suppress the production of interleukin-1.

Learning Response B: Incorrect. Glucocorticoids can act as a negative feedback because they suppress immune responses and suppress the production of interleukin-1.

Learning Response C: Incorrect. IL-1 synthesis is suppressed.

Learning Response D: Incorrect. Glucocorticoids suppress T cells and hence cell-mediated immunity.

Learning Response E: Incorrect. Glucocorticoids suppress T_{h1} cells and hence interferon-γ synthesis.

215. SUBJECT AREA: Effect of diet
QUESTION: Protein-calorie malnutrition does not affect:

- *A:* Lymphoid tissue
- *B:* The level of circulating CD4 T cells
- *C:* Cell-mediated immunity
- *D:* The affinity of antibody responses
- *E:* Phagocytosis of bacteria

☐ Correct Answer: *E*

Learning Response A: Incorrect. Lymphoid tissues are widely atrophied.

Learning Response B: Incorrect. Up to 50% reduction in circulating CD4 T cells often observed.

Learning Response C: Incorrect. Lack of CD4 cells produces seriously impaired cell-mediated immunity.

Learning Response D: Incorrect.

Learning Response E: Correct. Although intracellular destruction of bacteria after phagocytosis may be defective.

---

216. SUBJECT AREA: Effect of stress
QUESTION: The stress induced by severe exercise can increase susceptibility to infection by:

    A: Raising plasma levels of cortisol
    B: Increasing lymph flow
    C: Increasing synthesis of adrenaline
    D: Damaging mast cells
    E: Increasing the respiratory rate

☐ Correct Answer: *A*

Learning Response A: Correct. Cortisol depresses a range of immune responses.

Learning Response B: Incorrect.

Learning Response C: Incorrect.

Learning Response D: Incorrect.

Learning Response E: Incorrect.

---

217. SUBJECT AREA: Core revision
QUESTION: The level of antigen:

    A: Is unrelated to the intensity of the immune response
    B: Is related to the intensity of the immune response
    C: Never has an effect on the response to a T-independent antigen
    D: Has no effect on the concentration of MHC bound processed antigen
    E: Is constant in the extracellular fluid

☐ Correct Answer: *B*

Learning Response A: Incorrect. The lymphocyte responses are directly related to the availability of antigen.

Learning Response B: Correct. Lymphocytes are essentially driven by antigen and therefore the level determines the intensity of the immune response. The production of 'natural' antibodies is largely unrelated to stimulation by external antigen but is perhaps more based upon idiotypic interactions.

Learning Response C: Incorrect. T-independent antigens act by cross-linking surface receptors on B cells and the effect is therefore directly antigen concentration related.

Learning Response D: Incorrect. The concentration of MHC bound processed antigen will directly influence the drive of T lymphocytes by antigen-presenting cells.

Learning Response E: Incorrect. The antigen is constantly undergoing catabolism in the body.

218.
SUBJECT AREA: Core revision
QUESTION: IgG antibodies:

- *A:* Are the earliest class to appear in an immune response
- *B:* Are normally dimeric in mucosal secretions
- *C:* Remain of low affinity
- *D:* Inhibit antibody responses through the Fcγ receptor on B cells
- *E:* Augment antibody responses through the Fcγ receptor on B cells

☐ Correct Answer: *D*

Learning Response A: Incorrect. IgM is the earliest class to appear.

Learning Response B: Incorrect. The main immunoglobulin in mucosal secretions is dimeric IgA. When it occurs, IgG will be monomeric.

Learning Response C: Incorrect. IgG antibodies tend to be T-cell driven, and the high rate of mutation which occurs in these responses within germinal centers leads to selection of ever-increasing affinities.

Learning Response D: Correct. A complex between IgG antibody and antigen will cross-link surface immunoglobulin and Fcγ receptor on the B cell and cause inhibition.

Learning Response E: Incorrect. A complex between IgG antibody and antigen will cross-link surface immunoglobulin and Fcγ receptor on the B cell and cause inhibition.

219. SUBJECT AREA: Core revision
QUESTION: Suppressor T cells:

- *A:* Are always CD8
- *B:* Are always CD4
- *C:* May be T_{h2} cells suppressing T_{h1} by IL-4 or IL-10
- *D:* Do not exist
- *E:* Cannot transfer suppression to another animal

☐ Correct Answer: *C*

Learning Response A: Incorrect. Suppression can be obtained with CD4 cells.

Learning Response B: Incorrect. Suppression can be obtained with CD8 cells.

Learning Response C: Correct. T_{h1} and T_{h2} cells can be mutually suppressive and interferon-γ produced by T_{h1} can suppress T_{h2}.

Learning Response D: Incorrect. Operationally, T-cells can induce suppression. What has been questioned is the existence of cells dedicated just to suppression. For example, T_{h2} cells can suppress T_{h1} but will themselves functionally act to help B cells make antibody.

Learning Response E: Incorrect.

220. SUBJECT AREA: Core revision
QUESTION: Idiotype–anti-idiotype interactions:

- *A:* Do not involve antigen-specific receptors
- *B:* Only involve antibodies
- *C:* Can mediate a lymphocyte network in early life
- *D:* Do not occur within the CD5+ B-cell population
- *E:* Do not involve self-reactivity

☐ Correct Answer: *C*

Learning Response A: Incorrect. Idiotype and anti-idiotype interactions are similar to the involvement of variable regions of immunoglobulins with antigens.

Learning Response B: Incorrect. T cells can participate through their specific antigen receptors in idiotype networks.

Learning Response C: Correct. Hybridomas produced from neonatal spleens show a high percentage of mutual idiotypic interactions.

Learning Response D: Incorrect. This early network is particularly marked within the murine $CD5^+$ B-cell population.

Learning Response E: Incorrect. The reaction of an idiotype with an anti-idiotype is a self-reaction in the sense of reacting with another self-component in the body. The early idiotype network includes immunoglobulins, a high percentage of which will react with tissue autoantigens.

---

221. SUBJECT AREA: Control of immune responses
QUESTION: An immunoglobulin idiotype:

- *A:* Is defined by the antigen it reacts with
- *B:* Is defined by its anti-idiotype
- *C:* Is an isotypic variant
- *D:* Is an allotypic variant
- *E:* Is created by the C_{H1}/C_L domains

☐ Correct Answer: *B*

Learning Response A: Incorrect. The antibody is defined by its antigen.

Learning Response B: Correct. The idiotype is a feature of the antibody variable region, usually the hypervariable regions, which is recognized by an antibody or antiserum which reacts with those structures. Thus idiotype and anti-idiotype are mutually defining.

Learning Response C: Incorrect. Isotypic variants are present in the constant regions of Ig and are all present within the immunoglobulins of a normal individual. For example, an immunoglobulin class is an isotypic variant.

Learning Response D: Incorrect. Allotypic variants on immunoglobulins are polymorphic features which result from the use of alternative genes or of alleles.

Learning Response E: Incorrect. The idiotype is created by the variable domains.

222.
SUBJECT AREA: Core revision
QUESTION: High antibody responses linked to MHC class II genes:

- A: Are independent of MHC haplotype
- B: Depend on good T-helper cell recognition of class II/antigen peptide complex
- C: Depend on defective antigen presentation by MHC molecules
- D: Result from tolerance to MHC/self-peptide complexes
- E: Require suppression of T_{h2} cells

☐ Correct Answer: *B*

Learning Response A: Incorrect. The response varies with the MHC allele.

Learning Response B: Correct. The high antibody response requires a good T-helper activity which will depend upon effective recognition of the class II antigen peptide complex.

Learning Response C: Incorrect. Defective presentation by MHC will lead to poor T-helpers.

Learning Response D: Incorrect. Tolerance to MHC self-peptide may delete T-helpers not provide them.

Learning Response E: Incorrect. The suppression of T_{h2} cells is suppression of cells helping antibody responses.

223.
SUBJECT AREA: Core revision
QUESTION: With respect to immunoneuroendocrine networks:

- A: They do not exist
- B: They exist only in higher primates
- C: They cannot exist in subjects with a severed spinal cord
- D: Never involve the hypothalamic/pituitary axis
- E: Augmentation of glucocorticoid production by IL-1 is a good example

☐ Correct Answer: *E*

Learning Response A: Incorrect.

Learning Response B: Incorrect. They have been demonstrated in rodents and probably exist in most vertebrate species.

Learning Response C: Incorrect. The normal spinal reflex is probably not involved in most of these immunoneuroendocrine phenemona.

Learning Response D: Incorrect.

Learning Response E: Correct. IL-1 acts through the hypothalamus and pituitary to increase ACTH production which acts on the adrenal to augment glucocorticoids which suppress immune responses.

224.
SUBJECT AREA: Core revision
QUESTION: Cell-mediated immunity:

- *A:* Is unaffected by exercise
- *B:* Is unaffected by surgical trauma
- *C:* Is unaffected by diet
- *D:* May be grossly impaired by protein-calorie malnutrition
- *E:* Is unaffected by protein-calorie malnutrition

☐ Correct Answer: *D*

Learning Response A: Incorrect. Exercise induces stress and raises glucocorticoid levels which particularly affect T_{h1} cells concerned in cell-mediated immunity.

Learning Response B: Incorrect. Surgical trauma produces stress and the damage of tissues releases the immunosuppressive prostaglandin E_2.

Learning Response C: Incorrect. In protein-calorie malnutrition there is a profound reduction of CD4 cells and hence cell-mediated immunity.

Learning Response D: Correct. In protein-calorie malnutrition there is a profound reduction of CD4 cells and hence cell-mediated immunity.

Learning Response E: Incorrect. In protein-calorie malnutrition there is a profound reduction of CD4 cells and hence cell-mediated immunity.

225. SUBJECT AREA: Stem cells
QUESTION: Which of the following is the earliest site of hematopoiesis in the embryo:

    A: Bone marrow
    B: Liver
    C: Spleen
    D: Yolk sac
    E: Thymus

☐ Correct Answer: *D*

Learning Response A: Incorrect. The bone marrow is the major site of hematopoiesis from the noenatal period onwards.

Learning Response B: Incorrect. The liver is a major site of hematopoiesis in the embryo, but it is not the earliest site. Pro-B cells are present in fetal liver by 8-9 weeks of gestation in man and 14 days in the mouse.

Learning Response C: Incorrect. Hematopoiesis does occur in fetal spleen, but it is not the earliest site.

Learning Response D: Correct. Hematopoiesis originates in the early yolk sac but as embryogenesis proceeds this function is taken over by the fetal liver and then later by the bone marrow where it continues throughout life.

Learning Response E: Incorrect. The thymus is not a site of hematopoiesis but is the major site of T-cell development.

226. SUBJECT AREA: Stem cells
QUESTION: Stem cell factor is produced mainly by:

    A: Stem cells
    B: Thymic epithelium
    C: Bone marrow stromal cells
    D: Megakaryocytes
    E: The reticuloendothelial system

☐ Correct Answer: *C*

Learning Response A: Incorrect. Stem cell factor (SCF) acts on stem cells to guide their differentiation.

Learning Response B: Incorrect. The thymus produces various thymic hormones such as thymulin, thymopoietin, α_1-thymosin and β_4 thymosin.

Learning Response C: Correct. The bone marrow stromal cells comprise a complex mixture of cells including fibroblasts, macrophages and various other cell types. Stem cell factor (SCF) remains associated with the extracellular matrix and acts on primitive stem cells through a tyrosine kinase membrane receptor.

Learning Response D: Incorrect. The major function of magakaryocytes is to produce platelets.

Learning Response E: Incorrect. The reticuloendothelial system (RES) refers to the network of phagocytic and endothelial cells throughout the body.

227. SUBJECT AREA: Stem cells
QUESTION: The putative murine stem cell is positive for:

A: B220
B: Mac-1
C: Gr-1
D: CD8
E: Sca-1

☐ Correct Answer: *E*

Learning Response A: Incorrect. B220 is a B-cell marker.

Learning Response B: Incorrect. Mac-1 is a macrophage marker.

Learning Response C: Incorrect. Gr-1 is a granulocyte (polymorphonuclear leukocyte) marker.

Learning Response D: Incorrect. CD8 is a marker for cytotoxic T lymphocytes (CTL), whereas CD4 is a marker for helper T lymphocytes. This correlation holds up reasonably well, although the real relationship is with MHC recognition; $CD4^+$ T cells recognize MHC class II–bearing cells, whereas $CD8^+$ T cells recognize MHC class I–bearing cells.

Learning Response E: Correct. A monoclonal antibody recognises this 'stem cell antigen-1,' a cell surface antigen on putative murine stem cells. The putative marker for human stem cells is CD34.

---

228. SUBJECT AREA: The thymus
QUESTION: An example of a peptide hormone produced by the thymus is:

> A: Thymulin
> B: Thyroglobulin
> C: Thyroxine
> D: Thy-1
> E: Thymine

☐ Correct Answer: A

Learning Response A: Correct. Other peptide hormones secreted by the thymus are α_1-thymosin, β_4-thymosin and thymopoietin, although only thymulin and thymopoietin are exclusively of thymic origin.

Learning Response B: Incorrect. Thyroglobulin is the major glycoprotein in the thyroid gland and forms the precursor structure for the synthesis of thyroid hormones. It is a major autoantigen in thyroid autoimmunity.

Learning Response C: Incorrect. Thyroxine, tetraiodothyronine (T4), is one of the thyroid hormones. These are concerned with controlling metabolic rate.

Learning Response D: Incorrect. Thy-1 is a cell surface antigen found mainly on T-cells and in the brain.

Learning Response E: Incorrect. Thymine is one of the pyrimidine bases used to produce the DNA nucleotides.

---

229. SUBJECT AREA: The thymus
QUESTION: Hassall's corpuscles are found in:

> A: Peripheral blood
> B: Bone marrow
> C: Spleen
> D: Thymus
> E: Peyer's patches

☐ Correct Answer: *D*

Learning Response A: Incorrect. Erythrocytes are sometimes called red blood corpuscles, but they have nothing to do with Hassall's corpuscles which are not found in peripheral blood.

Learning Response B: Incorrect. Hassall's corpuscles are not found in the bone marrow.

Learning Response C: Incorrect. The spleen is divided into red pulp and white pulp, the white pulp forming the periarteriolar lymphoid sheaths (PALS).

Learning Response D: Correct. Whorled, possibly degenerate, aggregates of epithelial cells form these highly characteristic structures found in the thymus.

Learning Response E: Incorrect. The Peyer's patches are areas of lymphoid tissue in the gut.

---

230. SUBJECT AREA: The thymus
QUESTION: Which of the following statements might not be true:

A: Pluripotent stem cells are produced in the bone marrow
B: In adults, the thymus is virtually non-existent
C: Thymocytes are educated in the thymus
D: Not all lymphocytes are leukocytes
E: Plasma cells are always derived from B lymphocytes

☐ Correct Answer: *B*

Learning Response A: Incorrect. Pluripotent stem cells arising in the bone marrow give rise to all the blood cells, i.e., all leukocytes, erythrocytes and platelets.

Learning Response B: Correct. Quite a large normal thymus can be found in adults at autopsy, while involution in other samples may be due to stress associated with illness before death.

Learning Response C: Incorrect. Thymocytes undergo positive selection for self-MHC recognition and negative selection for (self) antigen recognition in the thymus, processes known as thymic education. Note that the developing T cells undergoing negative selection will not be able to differentiate self from foreign antigen; it is simply that the vast majority of antigens expressed in the thymus will be self.

Learning Response D: Incorrect. All lymphocytes are leukocytes (white cells).

Learning Response E: Incorrect. A fully differentiated B cell which actively secretes antibody is called a plasma cell.

---

231. SUBJECT AREA: The thymus
QUESTION: In a thymectomized animal which is irradiated and reconstituted with bone marrow cells:

- *A:* The T-lymphocyte population is not restored
- *B:* The B-lymphocyte population is not restored
- *C:* All lymphocyte populations are restored
- *D:* None of the lymphocyte populations are restored
- *E:* Rapid death inevitably follows

☐ Correct Answer: *A*

Learning Response A: Correct. Immature lymphocytes which are destined to become T cells travel from the bone marrow to the thymus where they differentiate to immunocompetence and are educated to recognize peptides derived from foreign antigens presented by self MHC molecules. Thus, in a thymectomized animal this process cannot take place.

Learning Response B: Incorrect. Most B-cell maturation takes place in the bone marrow itself.

Learning Response C: Incorrect. B cells but not T-lymphocyte populations are restored in a thymectomized animal which is irradiated and reconstituted with bone marrow cells.

Learning Response D: Incorrect. B-lymphocyte populations are restored in a thymectomized animal which is irradiated and reconstituted with bone marrow cells.

Learning Response E: Incorrect. Unless only given a very mild dose of irradiation, rapid death would follow (irrespective of whether or not the animal was thymectomized) in an animal unless it is 'rescued' by reconstitution with bone marrow cells. This is because the rapidly dividing stem cells in the bone marrow are particularly susceptible to the effect of radiation and if the production of leukocytes and platelets is severely impaired the animal will die from infection and/or hemorrhage.

232. SUBJECT AREA: T-cell ontogeny
QUESTION: In the thymic medulla the majority of γδ T cells are:

> A: CD4$^+$CD8$^+$
> B: CD4$^+$CD8$^-$
> C: CD4$^-$CD8$^+$
> D: CD4$^-$CD8$^-$
> E: Surface Ig$^+$

☐ Correct Answer: *D*

Learning Response A: Incorrect. 'Double positive' γδ T cells do not seem to occur.

Learning Response B: Incorrect. CD4$^+$CD8$^-$ γδ T cells are rarely, if ever, seen.

Learning Response C: Incorrect. Only a minority of the γδ T cells in the thymic medulla have this phenotype.

Learning Response D: Correct. By far the vast majority of γδ T cells are 'double negative' CD4$^-$CD8$^-$.

Learning Response E: Incorrect. T cells do not bear surface immunoglobulin, which is the antigen receptor of the B cell.

---

233. SUBJECT AREA: T-cell ontogeny
QUESTION: NK cells have:

> A: Rearranged TCR αβ genes
> B: Rearranged TCR γδ genes
> C: Rearranged immunoglobulin genes
> D: CD3
> E: CD4

☐ Correct Answer: *D*

Learning Response A: Incorrect. NK cells have TCR γδ genes which remain in the germ line (unrearranged) configuration.

Learning Response B: Incorrect. NK cells have TCR γδ genes which remain in the germ line (unrearranged) configuration.

Learning Response C: Incorrect. In NK cells both the heavy and light chain immunoglobulin gene loci remain in the germ line (unrearranged) configuration.

Learning Response D: Correct. NK cells are $CD2^+$, $CD3^+$, $CD8^+$, IL-2 receptor γ, produce interferon γ, and are driven to proliferate by IL-2. They are probably related to T cells in some way, but exactly how remains unclear.

Learning Response E: Incorrect. NK cells are $CD4^-$. This cell surface marker is found on the subpopulation of T cells which recognize MHC class II molecules (mostly helper T cells). In human and rat, but not in the mouse, CD4 is also expressed by monocytes, macrophages and by some dendritic cells.

234. SUBJECT AREA: Core revision
QUESTION: The first antigen receptor-bearing cells to appear in the thymus in mouse are:

A: T-cell receptor $\alpha\beta^+$
B: T-cell receptor $\gamma\delta^+$
C: TdT^-
D: $RAG-1^-$
E: $CD3^-$

☐ Correct Answer: *B*

Learning Response A: Incorrect. $\alpha\beta$ TCR (TCR2)-bearing cells appear in the murine thymus by day 19.

Learning Response B: Correct. $\gamma\delta$ TCR (TCR1)-bearing cells appear in the murine thymus by day 15.

Learning Response C: Incorrect. The enzyme terminal deoxynucleotidyl transferase (TdT) is thought to be involved in the insertion of nucleotide sequences at the N-terminal region of D and J segments in order to increase the diversity of the T-cell receptor. T cells undergoing T-cell receptor gene rearrangement therefore express this enzyme.

Learning Response D: Incorrect. The expression of the recombinase activator genes RAG-1 and RAG-2 is required for the rearrangement of T-cell receptor genes and therefore the first antigen receptor-bearing cells to appear in the thymus express these genes.

Learning Response E: Incorrect. In all immunocompetent T cells the antigen receptor is noncovalently associated with the CD3 complex which transduces the antigen recognition signal to the inside of the cell.

---

235. SUBJECT AREA: T-cell ontogeny
QUESTION: CD8$^+$ T cells in gut epithelium:

- *A:* Are always generated in the thymus
- *B:* Can express $\alpha\alpha$ homodimer T-cell receptors
- *C:* May be inside nurse cells
- *D:* Recognise native antigen
- *E:* Recognise MHC class II molecules

☐ Correct Answer: *B*

Learning Response A: Incorrect. At least some of the CD8$^+$ T cells in gut epithelium are known to be generated extrathymically.

Learning Response B: Correct. The receptors on CD8$^+$ T cells in gut epithelium which are generated extrathymically are $\alpha\alpha$ homodimers, in contrast to the $\alpha\beta$ heterodimers of conventional thymic T cells.

Learning Response C: Incorrect. Nurse cells are found in the thymic cortex, not in the gut epithelium. Thymocytes are found within the nurse cells, although their function (if any) in T-cell development is unclear.

Learning Response D: Incorrect. Unlike B cells, T cells do not recognize native antigen but recognize peptides derived from proteolytically-cleaved ('processed') antigen.

Learning Response E: Incorrect. CD8$^+$ T cells recognize MHC class I; it is CD4$^+$ T cells which recognize MHC class II.

---

236. SUBJECT AREA: T-cell ontogeny
QUESTION: Fetal $\alpha\beta$ T cells tend to use:

- *A:* V genes at random
- *B:* A single V gene
- *C:* V genes obtained by sister chromatid exchange
- *D:* The more 5' V genes
- *E:* The more 3' V genes

☐ Correct Answer: *E*

Learning Response A: Incorrect. There is a biased usage of αβ T-cell receptor genes by fetal T cells.

Learning Response B: Incorrect. Although fetal αβ T cells use a number of different V genes, virtually all of the first wave of fetal γδ T cells leaving the thymus in the mouse express the same V gene and colonize the skin. The second wave of fetal γδ T cells use the same δ gene combination but a different γ V-J pair and they seed the female reproductive organs.

Learning Response C: Incorrect. Fetal αβ T cells do not generally use V genes obtained by sister chromatid exchange.

Learning Response D: Incorrect. A bias towards 5' V genes is seen in the adult, not in the fetus.

Learning Response E: Correct. Fetal T cells tend to use the more 3' V genes, together with 5' J segments. In contrast, adults utilize a broader spectrum with some bias towards 5' V and 3' J gene segments.

237. SUBJECT AREA: T-cell ontogeny
QUESTION: Allelic exclusion is not seen for:

- *A:* T-cell receptor α genes
- *B:* T-cell receptor β genes
- *C:* T-cell receptor γ genes
- *D:* T-cell receptor δ genes
- *E:* T-cell receptor gene D region segments

☐ Correct Answer: A

Learning Response A: Correct. The α chains are not allelically excluded, so many cells can have two antigen-specific receptors each with their own α chain but sharing a common β chain.

Learning Response B: Incorrect. Following successful rearrangement on one allele, further rearrangement of Vβ genes on the sister chromatid is suppressed. Thus each cell expresses a single T-cell receptor β chain.

Learning Response C: Incorrect. Following successful rearrangement on one allele, further rearrangement of Vγ genes on the sister chromatid is suppressed.

Thus each cell expresses a single T-cell receptor γ chain.

Learning Response D: Incorrect. Following successful rearrangement on one allele, further rearrangement of Vδ genes on the sister chromatid is suppressed. Thus each cell expresses a single T-cell receptor δ chain.

Learning Response E: Incorrect. Following successful rearrangement on one allele, further rearrangement of most T-cell receptor genes on the sister chromatid is suppressed. This applies to three out of the four different types of T-cell receptor chain, but the exception lacks D region segments and therefore D segments are allelically excluded. Now you have a clue to the correct answer!

238. SUBJECT AREA: T-cell ontogeny
QUESTION: The first wave of fetal γδ T-cell receptor cells in mouse colonize the:

   A: Female reproductive tract
   B: Skin
   C: Peripheral blood
   D: Thymus
   E: Gut

☐ Correct Answer: *B*

Learning Response A: Incorrect. However, the second wave of fetal γδ T-cell receptor cells in mouse do colonize the female reproductive tract.

Learning Response B: Correct. Nearly all γδ T cells in the skin express the same variable region gene, Vγ5 and Vδ1.

Learning Response C: Incorrect. γδ T cells in the peripheral blood are, like other lymphocytes, *in transit* to the sites of immune responses.

Learning Response D: Incorrect. As with αβ T cells, γδ T cells leave the thymus, but do not colonize it.

Learning Response E: Incorrect. In the adult mouse, intraepithelial γδ T cells in the intestine predominantly express Vγ7, whereas those in the spleen, lymph nodes and blood predominantly express Vγ4. However, unlike fetal γδ T cells, adult receptors show a high degree of junctional diversity.

239. SUBJECT AREA: T-cell ontogeny

QUESTION: In human adult peripheral blood the percentage of γδ T cells bearing Vγ9, Vδ2 T-cell receptors is:

A: <1%
B: 25%
C: 50%
D: <30%
E: 70%

☐ Correct Answer: *E*

Learning Response A: Incorrect. There are many more than this!

Learning Response B: Incorrect. This is the percentage of Vγ9, Vδ2 T cells in cord blood.

Learning Response C: Incorrect. This is the percentage of Vγ1, Vδ2 TCR-bearing cells in cord blood.

Learning Response D: Incorrect. This is the percentage of Vγ1, Vδ2 TCR-bearing cells in adult blood.

Learning Response E: Correct. The percentage rises to this figure from around 25% in cord blood.

---

240. SUBJECT AREA: T-cell ontogeny

QUESTION: The T cells in male H-2^b SCID mice bearing a transgenic αβ T-cell receptor gene specific for H-Y in association with H-2D^b will:

A: All be CD4$^+$CD8$^-$
B: All be CD4$^-$CD8$^+$
C: All recognise H-Y
D: Undergo continuous proliferation
E: Be deleted

☐ Correct Answer: *E*

Learning Response A: Incorrect. H-2D is a class I MHC molecule and therefore would not select CD4$^+$ cells.

Learning Response B: Incorrect. These could be selected in female mice, but not in male mice.

Learning Response C: Incorrect. Try again!

Learning Response D: Incorrect. These T cells will not undergo continuous proliferation in this environment.

Learning Response E: Correct. H-Y is the male antigen. SCID mice have a normal thymus and therefore the transgenic T cells will undergo negative selection upon encounter with the self antigen H-Y presented by self MHC H-2D^b.

---

241. SUBJECT AREA: T-cell tolerance
QUESTION: In Sir Peter Medawar's experiments demonstrating the development of immunological tolerance:

A: Thymectomized mice had to be used
B: SCID mice were used
C: The mice were chimeric
D: Skin grafts were always rejected
E: Tolerance could not be induced in neonatal mice

☐ Correct Answer: *C*

Learning Response A: Incorrect. Note, however, the role of the thymus. Since recruitment of newly competent T cells is drastically curtailed by removal of the thymus, the tolerant state persists for much longer in thymectomized animals.

Learning Response B: Incorrect. Severe combined immunodeficient (SCID) mice were not generally available forty years ago at the time of Sir Peter Medawar's experiments and, in any case, the controls would be unresponsive to grafts because they had no immunocompetent lymphocytes.

Learning Response C: Correct. CBA cells were injected neonatally into A strain mice and because a state of tolerance is established the injected CBA cells survived and the animals continue to be chimeric. In this case the tolerance is long term, but with non-living antigens such as bovine serum albumin (BSA) tolerance is gradually lost, probably due to new immunocompetent cells developing following the catabolism of the antigen.

Learning Response D: Incorrect. These experiments were aimed at inducing immunological tolerance such that skin grafts from a different strain would no longer be seen as foreign and therefore would not be rejected.

Learning Response E: Incorrect. Tolerance usually was induced in neonatal mice, which are generally easier to tolerize than adults.

242. SUBJECT AREA: Core revision
QUESTION: Positive selection in the thymus is thought to be mediated by:

    A: Thymic epithelial cells
    B: Macrophages
    C: Dendritic cells
    D: B cells
    E: T cells

☐ Correct Answer: *A*

Learning Response A: Correct. Cortical epithelial cells may be relatively inefficient antigen processors and only deliver a weak signal which induces proliferation rather than deletion of immature thymocytes.

Learning Response B: Incorrect. Macrophages in the thymus are probably primarily concerned with tolerance induction to self (i.e., negative selection).

Learning Response C: Incorrect. Dendritic cells in the thymus are probably primarily concerned with tolerance induction to self (i.e., negative selection).

Learning Response D: Incorrect. There are a few B cells in the thymus and these may also be primarily concerned with tolerance induction to self (i.e., negative selection).

Learning Response E: Incorrect. It is the T cells themselves which are positively selected for recognition of self MHC molecules.

243. SUBJECT AREA: Core revision
QUESTION: B1 cells are:

    A: B cells which respond to mostly to T-dependent antigens
    B: B cells which predominate in later life
    C: Plasma cells
    D: $CD5^-$ B cells
    E: $CD5^+$ B cells

☐ Correct Answer: *E*

Learning Response A: Incorrect. B1 cells tend to respond to T-independent antigens.

Learning Response B: Incorrect. B1 cells predominate in early life.

Learning Response C: Incorrect. Both B1 and B2 cells become plasma cells when fully differentiated, although the spectrum of antibodies secreted by these two populations is different.

Learning Response D: Incorrect. $CD5^-$ B cells are the major B-cell population and are referred to as B2 cells.

Learning Response E: Correct. $CD5^+$ B cells are referred to as B1 cells. They are a minor population and predominate in early life when they show a high level of idiotype–anti-idiotype connectivity, and produce low affinity polyreactive IgM antibodies many of which are autoantibodies.

244.
SUBJECT AREA: Core revision
QUESTION: V_{preB} :

- *A:* Refers to all the germ line immunoglobulin heavy chain V genes in the pre-B cell
- *B:* Is part of the surrogate light chain
- *C:* Forms a structure with $\lambda 3$
- *D:* Forms a structure with $C\kappa$
- *E:* Is expressed by both T and B cells

☐ Correct Answer: *B*

Learning Response A: Incorrect. There are about eighty immunoglobulin heavy chain germ line V genes in a pre-B cell, but these are not called V_{preB}.

Learning Response B: Correct. Together with λ_5, V_{preB} associates with μ heavy chain to generate a surrogate 'IgM' receptor. Expression of this receptor is absolutely required for further differentiation of the B cell.

Learning Response C: Incorrect. $\lambda 3$ is one of the conventional λ light chain constant region genes and does not associate with V_{preB}.

Learning Response D: Incorrect. Unlike the λ light chain locus, in the κ chain locus there is only a single $C\kappa$. This does not associate with V_{preB}.

Learning Response E: Incorrect. V_{preB} is not expressed on T cells, only on immature B cells.

245. SUBJECT AREA: Core revision
QUESTION: Which of the following molecules does not belong to the Ig gene superfamily:

      A: Immunoglobulin
      B: T-cell receptor
      C: β_2-microglobulin
      D: Thy-1
      E: LFA-1

☐ Correct Answer: *E*

Learning Response A: Incorrect. Immunoglobulin is the prototype of the Ig gene superfamily. The success of the immunoglobulin domain structure in allowing non-covalent mutual interactions between proteins is reflected in the very large number of diverse recognition molecules which belong to this superfamily.

Learning Response B: Incorrect. Both the $\gamma\delta$ and the $\alpha\beta$ T-cell receptors belong to the immunoglobulin gene superfamily.

Learning Response C: Incorrect. β_2-microglobulin, the nonpolymorphic molecule which is noncovalently associated with the polymorphic MHC class I α chain, is composed of a single Ig-type domain. The α chain of MHC class I consists of three extracellular domains, the most membrane-proximal of which is a member of the Ig gene superfamily.

Learning Response D: Incorrect. Thy-1 consists of a single domain which is a member of the Ig gene superfamily.

Learning Response E: Correct. LFA-1 is a member of the integrin family, molecules concerned with leukocyte binding to endothelial cells and to extracellular matrix proteins. The VLA molecules are also members of the integrin superfamily.

246. SUBJECT AREA: Core revision
QUESTION: Which immunoglobulin class crosses the placenta to provide a high level of passive immunity at birth:

A: IgA
B: IgD
C: IgE
D: IgG
E: IgM

☐ Correct Answer: *D*

Learning Response A: Incorrect. Secretory IgA is present in breast milk and will provide enteric protection for the newborn in breast-fed babies, but it is not transported across the placenta and does not enter the baby's circulation from the gut lumen.

Learning Response B: Incorrect. IgD is largely a cell surface-associated immunoglobulin which acts as an antigen receptor on the B lymphocyte. The small amount of IgD in the maternal circulation does not cross the placenta.

Learning Response C: Incorrect. IgE is normally only present at extremely low levels and does not cross the placenta.

Learning Response D: Correct. IgG is the only class of immunoglobulin which is acquired by the neonate by placental transfer from the mother. This process is dependent upon Fc structures specific to this Ig class. The maternal IgG is catabolized with a half-life of approximately 30 days.

Learning Response E: Incorrect. IgM does not cross the placenta. The low but significant levels of IgM in cord blood are synthesized by the baby and reach adult levels by nine months of age.

247. SUBJECT AREA: B-cell tolerance
QUESTION: Strains of mice which are congenitally deficient in C5:

A: Do not possess C5-responsive lymphocytes
B: Have both T and B cells that can respond to C5
C: Have T, but not B, cells that can respond to C5
D: Have B, but not T, cells that can respond to C5
E: Have C5-specific monocytes, but not lymphocytes

☐ Correct Answer: *B*

Learning Response A: Incorrect. Because this self antigen is never expressed in the mice, C5-responsive lymphocytes are not subjected to the normal tolerance mechanisms and are therefore able to enter the periphery.

Learning Response B: Correct. Because this self antigen is never expressed in these mice, neither the T cells nor the B cells are subjected to the normal tolerance mechanisms and they are both therefore able to enter the periphery.

Learning Response C: Incorrect. With soluble proteins at least, T cells are more readily tolerized than B cells. However, because C5 is never expressed in these mice, neither T cells nor B cells will be tolerized.

Learning Response D: Incorrect. Normal mice, not C5-deficient mice, have B but not T lymphocytes that can respond to C5. With soluble proteins at least, T cells are more readily tolerized than B cells. Thus, C5-reactive B cells are normally present in the body but cannot be triggered by this T-dependent self antigen since the T cells required to provide the necessary T-B help are tolerant.

Learning Response E: Incorrect. Only lymphocytes show antigen specificity, not monocytes. This is because lymphocytes are the only cells to express a clonally-restricted antigen receptor, antibody in the case of B cells and the T cell receptor in the case of T cells.

248. SUBJECT AREA: B-cell ontogeny
QUESTION: The phenomenon whereby, following successful Ig gene rearrangement, further rearrangement on the sister chromatid is suppressed is called:

   A: Allelic exclusion
   B: Class switching
   C: Productive rearrangement
   D: Clonal selection
   E: Gene shuffling

☐ Correct Answer: A

Learning Response A: Correct. All of the immunoglobulin gene loci (heavy, κ light, λ light) exhibit allelic exclusion, as do all of the T-cell receptor gene loci except the α chain. Thus a B-cell is able to express only one light and one heavy chain specificity.

Learning Response B: Incorrect. Class switching only occurs on the chromatid on which successful VDJ rearrangement has occurred because heavy chain transcription requires constant regions in the cis as distinct from the trans configuration, and without a successful rearrangement of these genes the antibody cannot be expressed.

Learning Response C: Incorrect. A successful immunoglobulin gene rearrangement is, by definition, a productive rearrangement and this will suppress any further rearrangement at that locus. A non-productive rearrangement would be one in which adjacent segments are joined in an incorrect reading frame or in such a way as to generate a termination codon downstream from the splice point. In this case a second attempt at rearrangement can be undertaken on the sister chromatid.

Learning Response D: Incorrect. The expression of only one light chain and one heavy chain is essential for clonal selection to operate since this cell is then only programmed to make the one antibody. This it uses as its cell surface receptor to recognize antigen.

Learning Response E: Incorrect. The term gene shuffling is sometimes used to describe the process of selecting one gene segment from each of the pool of V, D and J gene segments used to make an antigen receptor using gene rearrangement.

249. SUBJECT AREA: Evolution of the immune response
QUESTION: Genuine adaptive T- and B-cell responses are seen in:

    A: The Californian hagfish
    B: The horseshoe crab
    C: *Xenopus*
    D: *Botryllus schosseri*
    E: Earthworms

☐ Correct Answer: *C*

Learning Response A: Incorrect. Neither T- nor B-cell responses can be elicited in this cyclostome.

Learning Response B: Incorrect. In many phyla, phagocytosis is augmented by coating of antigen with agglutinins and bactericidins. The horseshoe crab possesses an α_2-macroglobulin structurally homologous to C3.

Learning Response C: Correct. The toad, *Xenopus*, has a less complex lymphoid system than mammals, characterized by a small number of lymphocytes and a restricted antibody repertoire which does not undergo somatic mutation. Note that both positive and negative thymic selection has been demonstrated in frogs.

Learning Response D: Incorrect. The colonial tunicate *Botryllus schosseri* is able to differentiate self from nonself. However, there is little evidence in these responses for allele-specific memory and it is questionable whether this and related phenomena in the lower animal orders are true precedents of T-cell-mediated reactions in vertebrates.

Learning Response E: Incorrect. Mechanisms for the recognition and subsequent rejection of nonself can be identified in invertebrates although they do not have lymphocytes. A xenograft of body wall tissue from the earthworm *Eisenia* onto the earthworm *Lumbricus* is completely destroyed by 50 days, whereas an autograft is accepted.

250. SUBJECT AREA: Cellular recognition molecules
QUESTION: A member of the immunoglobulin gene superfamily which contains 5 Ig-type domains is:

A: Thy-1
B: Poly-Ig receptor
C: N-CAM
D: CD4
E: CD3ε

☐ Correct Answer: *B*

Learning Response A: Incorrect. Thy-1 consists of a single Ig-type domain, and is present on T cells and neurons.

Learning Response B: Correct. The poly-Ig receptor consists of 5 Ig-type domains. It transports IgA across mucosal membranes.

Learning Response C: Incorrect. N-CAM possesses 4 Ig-type domains and is an adhesion molecule binding neuronal cells together.

Learning Response D: Incorrect. CD4 has one Ig-type domain and three other domains which do not belong to the Ig gene superfamily. It helps to focus the helper cell onto cells bearing MHC class II molecules.

Learning Response E: Incorrect. CD3ε has a single Ig-type domain. Together with CD3γ, CD3δ and the associated ζ and η molecules, it forms the signal transduction unit of the T-cell receptor.

251. SUBJECT AREA: Inflammation
QUESTION: Histamine:

A: Has no effect on the permeability of venules
B: Constricts arterioles
C: Upregulates adhesion molecules on vascular endothelium
D: Upregulates IL-8
E: Induces polymorph chemotaxis

☐ Correct Answer: *C*

Learning Response A: Incorrect. Histamine increases the permeability of venules.

Learning Response B: Incorrect. It dilates arterioles.

Learning Response C: Correct. Histamine upregulates P-selectin of vascular endothelium.

Learning Response D: Incorrect. IL-8 is upregulated later in the inflammatory response by TNFα, IL-1 or LPS.

Learning Response E: Incorrect.

252. SUBJECT AREA: Inflammation (p.244/5)
QUESTION: P-selectin pairs with:

A: LFA-3
B: LFA-1
C: ICAM-1
D: Sialyl Lewis^X
E: β_2 integrin molecules

☐ Correct Answer: *D*

Learning Response A: Incorrect. LFA-3 pairs with CD2.

Learning Response B: Incorrect. LFA-1 pairs with ICAM-1.

Learning Response C: Incorrect. ICAM-1 pairs with LFA-1.

Learning Response D: Correct.

Learning Response E: Incorrect. β_2 integrin molecules include LFA-1.

253.
SUBJECT AREA: Inflammation

QUESTION: Binding of platelet activating factor (PAF) to its receptor on the polymorph:

- A: Initiates binding of polymorphs to P-selectin
- B: Initiates polymorph rolling
- C: Produces a chemotactic gradient
- D: Causes histamine release
- E: Upregulates LFA-1

☐ Correct Answer: *E*

Learning Response A: Incorrect. Initiation of binding is by histamine and thrombin.

Learning Response B: Incorrect. The binding to P-selectin is what initiates rolling.

Learning Response C: Incorrect.

Learning Response D: Incorrect.

Learning Response E: Correct. The binding of PAF to its receptor on the PMN upregulates LFA-1 which now anchors the PMN firmly to ICAM-1 on the endothelial cell surface.

254.
SUBJECT AREA: Inflammation

QUESTION: Activated Hageman factor:

- A: Produces a fibrin clot in damaged veins
- B: Is factor X of the intrinsic clotting system
- C: Directly causes thrombus formation
- D: Directly increases vascular permeability
- E: Directly dissolves fibrin clots

☐ Correct Answer: *A*

Learning Response A: Correct. The Hageman factor activates the intrinsic clotting system which leads to thrombin activation and the splitting of fibrinogen into fibrin.

Learning Response B: Incorrect. Hageman factor is factor XI.

Learning Response C: Incorrect. Indirectly, activation of thrombin by Hageman factor can release platelet activating factor which induces thrombus formation. The thrombus is normally produced in the arterial system by platelet activation through contact with basement membrane collagen, LPS, or induced endothelial platelet activating factor.

Learning Response D: Incorrect. Inflammatory mediators increase vascular permeability which is a component of the inflammatory process.

Learning Response E: Incorrect. Fibrin is dissolved *indirectly* by plasmin activated by kalikrein, itself activated by Hageman factor.

255.
SUBJECT AREA: Inflammation
QUESTION: Polymorph chemotaxis is mediated by:

        A: C5b
        B: IL-8
        C: C3a
        D: MCP-1
        E: E-selectin

☐ Correct Answer: *B*

Learning Response A: Incorrect. C5b initiates the terminal membrane attack complex. The other C5 fragment, C5a, is a powerful chemotactic agent.

Learning Response B: Correct. IL-8 produced by endothelial cells later in the inflammatory response is a powerful chemotactic agent for polys.

Learning Response C: Incorrect. C3a is an anaphylatoxin which liberates histamine from mast cells.

Learning Response D: Incorrect. MCP-1 is a monocyte chemotactic protein produced by the action of IL-1 and TNFα on endothelial cells, fibroblasts and epithelial cells.

Learning Response E: Incorrect. E-selectin is a late inflammatory adhesion molecule which binds and activates neutrophils.

256. SUBJECT AREA: Inflammation
QUESTION: Opsonization of bacteria occurs through coating bacteria just with:

A: C3b
B: C5a
C: Membrane attack complex
D: F(ab')$_2$ IgG
E: IgM

☐ Correct Answer: *A*

Learning Response A: Correct. There are receptors for C3b on the surface of phagocytic cells.

Learning Response B: Incorrect. There are no surface receptors for C5a which also does not bind to bacteria. It is a powerful anaphylatoxin and chemotactic molecule.

Learning Response C: Incorrect. The membrane attack complex C5b–C9 inserts into the membrane and causes cytotoxicity.

Learning Response D: Incorrect. F(ab)'$_2$ lacks the Fc region which would enable the bacteria to bind to the Fcγ receptors on phagocytic cells.

Learning Response E: Incorrect. There are no receptors for IgM on the phagocytic cells although coating of bacteria with IgM would lead to complement activation and opsonization through C3b.

257. SUBJECT AREA: Inflammation
QUESTION: The inflammatory process resolves under the influence of:

A: PGE$_2$
B: TGFβ
C: Glucocorticoids
D: All the above
E: None of the above

☐ Correct Answer: *D*

Learning Response A: True but not as correct as D.

Learning Response B: True but not as correct as D.

Learning Response C: True but not as correct as D.

Learning Response D: Correct.

Learning Response E: Incorrect.

---

258. SUBJECT AREA: Inflammation
QUESTION: A granuloma formed by chronic inflammation:

- *A:* Walls off a persisting agent
- *B:* Is characterized by polymorphs
- *C:* Is characterized by macrophages
- *D:* Involves A & B
- *E:* Involves A & C

☐ Correct Answer: *E*

Learning Response A: True but not as correct as E.

Learning Response B: Incorrect.

Learning Response C: True but not as correct as E.

Learning Response D: Incorrect.

Learning Response E: Correct.

---

259. SUBJECT AREA: Inflammation
QUESTION: Extracellular bacteria are optimally killed by:

- *A:* Polymorphs
- *B:* Complement
- *C:* Antibody
- *D:* Macrophages plus complement
- *E:* Polymorphs plus antibody plus complement

☐ Correct Answer: *E*

Learning Response A: Incorrect.

Learning Response B: Incorrect.

Learning Response C: Incorrect.

Learning Response D: Incorrect.

Learning Response E: Correct. Bacteria opsonized by IgG and C3b will adhere and activate polymorphs for phagocytosis and killing.

260. SUBJECT AREA: Killing extracellular bacteria
QUESTION: Extracellular bacteria try to avoid killing by:

   A: Activating polymorphs
   B: Accelerating complement activation
   C: Synthesizing capsules
   D: Deviating complement deposition to the cell membrane
   E: Limiting variation in their antigens

☐ Correct Answer: *C*

Learning Response A: Incorrect. This would accelerate killing. Exotoxins secreted by bacteria can poison polymorphs.

Learning Response B: Incorrect. This would accelerate bacterial death. Bacteria accelerates complement breakdown by binding factor H which helps cleavage of C3b by factor I. Other bacteria produce molecules which mimic complement degrading proteins.

Learning Response C: Correct. Capsules do not adhere readily to phagocytic cells and may cover carbohydrate molecules which could be recognized by phagocyte receptors.

Learning Response D: Incorrect. The complement deposition on the cell membrane would help to cause death of the bacterium. Deviation is usually to sites distant from the cell membrane, e.g., on the terminii of flagellii.

Learning Response E: Incorrect. Variation in bacterial antigens helps their survival in the face of immune attack.

261. SUBJECT AREA: Extracellular bacteria
QUESTION: Toxins are neutralized by:

   A: Complement
   B: Antibody
   C: Toxoids
   D: Polymorphs
   E: Proteolytic enzymes

☐ Correct Answer: *B*

Learning Response A: Incorrect. Toxins do not normally directly activate the complement system.

Learning Response B: Correct. Antibody may block the binding to target cell and would increase the rate of removal of toxin from the circulation by immune complex formation.

Learning Response C: Incorrect. Toxoids are altered toxins which are biologically inactive but induce protective immune responses as vaccines.

Learning Response D: Incorrect.

Learning Response E: Incorrect. Although proteolytic enzymes can degrade toxins, the speed of this reaction within the body would be too slow to contribute significantly to protection.

262. SUBJECT AREA: Extracellular bacteria
QUESTION: CR1 complement receptors on phagocytic cells bind:

   A: Factor H
   B: Factor I
   C: C3d
   D: Inactive C3b (iC3b)
   E: C3b

☐ Correct Answer: *E*

Learning Response A: Incorrect. Factor H binds to C3b.

Learning Response B: Incorrect. Factor I cleaves the factor H C3b complex.

Learning Response C: Incorrect. C3d binds to CR2 receptors.

Learning Response D: Incorrect. iC3b binds to CR3 receptors.

Learning Response E: Correct.

---

263. SUBJECT AREA: Extracellular bacteria
QUESTION: Secretory IgA protects external mucosal surfaces by:

      A: Firing mast cells
      B: Recruiting phagocytic cells
      C: Preventing microbial adherence to the mucosa
      D: Binding to epithelial cells
      E: Its secretory piece

☐ Correct Answer: *C*

Learning Response A: Incorrect. Mast cells are fired in particular either by IgE cross-linking on their surface through antigen, or through the anaphylatoxins C5a and C3a.

Learning Response B: Incorrect. Phagocytic cells are recruited by chemotactic agents such as IL-8 and C5a.

Learning Response C: Correct. The IgA blocks adherence of bacteria to the mucosa and also facilitates opsonization through binding to Fcα receptors on phagocytic cells.

Learning Response D: Incorrect. There is little evidence for significant binding to epithelial cells.

Learning Response E: Incorrect. The secretory piece protects IgA from proteolytic breakdown.

---

264. SUBJECT AREA: Extracellular bacteria
QUESTION: The pyrogenic streptococcal exotoxins SPE, A, B and C:

      A: Are M proteins
      B: Cause post-streptococcal autoimmune disease

    C: Produce high titers of anti-streptolysin O
    D: Have hyaluronidase activity
    E: Are superantigens

☐ Correct Answer: *E*

Learning Response A: Incorrect. M proteins are structural proteins of the streptococcus which induce strong protective immunity.

Learning Response B: Incorrect. Antigens which cross-react with heart muscle are thought to be responsible for inducing the autoimmune disease.

Learning Response C: Incorrect. Streptolysin O is a different antigen.

Learning Response D: Incorrect. Certain exotoxins have this enzyme activity thereby facilitating spread of the bacterial infection.

Learning Response E: Correct. The superantigens combine with the framework regions of certain Vβ families irrespective of their complementarity determining regions which are specific for particular T-cell epitopes.

265.
SUBJECT AREA: Extracellular bacteria
QUESTION: *Neisseria* infection is more serious in individuals lacking:

    A: Gut flora
    B: Gastric pepsin
    C: Factor B
    D: C8 or C9
    E: IgG

☐ Correct Answer: D

Learning Response A: Incorrect.

Learning Response B: Incorrect.

Learning Response C: Incorrect.

Learning Response D: Correct. The membrane attack complex containing C8 and C9 is important for destroying the *Neisseria* bacterium.

Learning Response E: Incorrect.

266. SUBJECT AREA: Intracellular bacteria
QUESTION: Specific immunity to *M. tuberculosis* in mice can be transferred to naive histocompatible recipients by:

A: B cells
B: T cells
C: Macrophages
D: Polymorphs
E: IgG

☐ Correct Answer: *B*

Learning Response A: Incorrect. Antibodies do not provide immunity to *M. tuberculosis*.

Learning Response B: Correct. T cells are important for immunity to *M. tuberculosis* through the provision of T_{h1} cytokines to activate macrophages containing the bacilli and perhaps also the participation of cytotoxic T cells. The latter may kill macrophages which cannot be rescued by cytokines thereby releasing the bacteria to be taken up by fresh young macrophages which can be activated to become killers.

Learning Response C: Incorrect. Although macrophages are the final killers of the bacilli, without T-cell help they are silenced by intracellular infection with this organism.

Learning Response D: Incorrect. Polymorphs are not involved in any way.

Learning Response E: Incorrect.

267. SUBJECT AREA: Intracellular bacteria
QUESTION: Lepromatous leprosy is characterized by:

A: Poor T-cell responses
B: Good cell-mediated immunity
C: Good lepromin dermal response
D: Poor B-cell responses
E: Poor phagocytic ability

☐ Correct Answer: *A*

Learning Response A: Correct. The poor T-cell responses specific for the leprosy bacillus prevents the host from mounting a killing response and the bacilli grow profusely.

Learning Response B: Incorrect.

Learning Response C: Incorrect. The poor dermal response to lepromin represents a deficient delayed hypersensitivity response.

Learning Response D: Incorrect.

Learning Response E: Incorrect.

268. SUBJECT AREA: Viral infection
QUESTION: Viral antigen *shift* involves:

        A: Single point mutation
        B: Random point mutations
        C: Interchange of large amounts of the viral genome with other viruses
        D: Rearrangement of the viral structural architecture
        E: Regression to an earlier variant

☐ Correct Answer: *C*

Learning Response A: Incorrect. Single point mutation leads to antigenic drift, so changing antigen specificity in a moderate way.

Learning Response B: Incorrect. These will lead to changes in antigen but are not normally referred to as antigenic shift.

Learning Response C: Correct. The ability to interchange large segments of the genome with a viral reservoir in other animal species is the basis of antigenic shift leading to radical change in antigen, particularly crucial antigens giving protective immunity such as the viral hemagglutinin.

Learning Response D: Incorrect. The rearrangement of surface antigens is a device used by certain parasites to evade the immune system.

Learning Response E: Incorrect.

269. SUBJECT AREA: Viral infection
QUESTION: Interferons:

      A: Opsonize viruses
      B: Neutralize viruses
      C: Play a major role in recovery from infection
      D: Prevent viral entry into cells
      E: Protect against reinfection

☐ Correct Answer: *C*

Learning Response A: Incorrect. Viruses are opsonized by antibody and complement.

Learning Response B: Incorrect. Viruses are neutralized largely by antibody.

Learning Response C: Correct. Interferon inhibits the intracellular replication of viruses.

Learning Response D: Incorrect. Prevention of entry may be effected by antibody.

Learning Response E: Incorrect. Protection against reinfection is largely mediated by antibody.

270. SUBJECT AREA: Viral infection
QUESTION: Cytotoxic T cells:

      A: Are usually CD4
      B: Recognize native viral antigen
      C: Are more readily produced by killed rather than live virus
      D: Kill viruses directly
      E: Restrict viral replication

☐ Correct Answer: *E*

Learning Response A: Incorrect. Cytotoxic cells are usually CD8. CD4 cells can sometimes be cytotoxic through secretion of cytokines such as TNF.

Learning Response B: Incorrect. T cells never recognize native, only processed antigens.

Learning Response C: Incorrect. The presentation of viral protein antigen in the processed form on the cell surface associated with MHC class I, is more frequent when the viral protein is present in the cytosol and passes through the normal class I transport processing mechanism.

Learning Response D: Incorrect. Cytotoxic T cells kill other cells.

Learning Response E: Correct. The early killing of a virally infected cell prevents the virus from utilizing that cell for replication.

271. SUBJECT AREA: Viral infection
QUESTION: NK cells:

    A: Have rearranged T-cell receptor genes
    B: Are unaffected by IFNα
    C: Are more active against targets with upregulated MHC class I
    D: Can kill certain virally-infected cells
    E: Can kill all virally-infected cells

☐ Correct Answer: *D*

Learning Response A: Incorrect. The T-cell receptor genes are not rearranged to produce an antigen-specific receptor. The receptors tend to be specific for groups of surface molecules such as carbohydrates.

Learning Response B: Incorrect. The NK cells are stimulated by interferon-α.

Learning Response C: Incorrect. The presence of class I tends to inhibit the action of NK cells.

Learning Response D: Correct. Like cytotoxic T cells, NK cells can inhibit viral replication by killing the host cell. The difference is that cytotoxic T cells have a receptor for a specific T-cell epitope whereas NK cells have a broader specificity.

Learning Response E: Incorrect. The recognition and killing of virally infected cells is restricted to certain of the viruses, presumably reflecting the lack of universal recognition by the NK cell receptors.

272. SUBJECT AREA: Parasitic infections
QUESTION: IgE levels are high in infections with:

A: *Trichinella spiralis*
B: *Trypanosoma cruzi*
C: *Trypanosoma rhodesiense*
D: *Plasmodium falciparum*
E: *Leishmania tropica*

☐ Correct Answer: A

Learning Response A: Correct. Parasites like *Trichinella* frequently increase the IgE levels, usually polyclonally. This tends to inhibit the protective effect of IgE by diluting out the specific IgE on the mast cell. Inflammation induced by mast cell degranulation leads to influx of IgG which causes damage to the parasite.

Learning Response B: Incorrect. This organism is killed by T-cell activation of macrophages.

Learning Response C: Incorrect. This organism is largely combatted by antibody.

Learning Response D: Incorrect. Protection, where it exists, is complex.

Learning Response E: Incorrect. This intracellular organism is killed by T-cell activation of macrophages.

273. SUBJECT AREA: Parasitic infections
QUESTION: T_{h1} cells are of major importance in defense against:

A: *Trypanosoma brucei*
B: *Leishmania donovani*
C: Malarial merozoites
D: All of the above
E: None of the above

☐ Correct Answer: B

Learning Response A: Incorrect. Antibodies provide the major defense.

Learning Response B: Correct. T_{h1} cells produce cytokines which activate the killing macrophages. Where T_{h2} cells predominate, antibodies are produced and the individual responds poorly to the infection.

Learning Response C: Incorrect. Mainly antibody-mediated protection.

Learning Response D: Incorrect. See learning responses A, B & C.

Learning Response E: Incorrect. See learning response B.

---

274. SUBJECT AREA: Parasitic infections
QUESTION: Trypanosomes evade the host immune response by:

- *A:* Pre-empting complement defenses
- *B:* Molecular mimicry of host antigens
- *C:* Varying their surface antigens
- *D:* Suppressing cell-mediated immunity
- *E:* Suppressing antibody production

☐ Correct Answer: *C*

Learning Response A: Incorrect. *T. cruzi* produces a DAF-like molecule which accelerates C3b decay.

Learning Response B: Incorrect. Ascaris antigens cross-react with human collagen and are thereby less immunogenic.

Learning Response C: Correct. The trypanosome produces a sequential array of host antigens which change as the host makes a good antibody response.

Learning Response D: Incorrect. Infection by *T. brucei* can suppress cell-mediated immunity.

Learning Response E: Incorrect. *T. brucei* can inhibit antibody production and T-suppressor activity is prominent.

---

275. SUBJECT AREA: Parasitic infections
QUESTION: Immune complex-induced nephrotic syndrome is a feature of:

- *A:* Trypanosomiasis
- *B:* Quartan malaria
- *C:* Schistosomiasis
- *D:* Leishmaniasis
- *E:* Filariasis

☐ Correct Answer: *B*

Learning Response A: Incorrect. Wasting of cattle with trypanosomiasis is due to increased TNF levels.

Learning Response B: Correct.

Learning Response C: Incorrect. The eggs induce liver damage from T-cell mediated granulomata.

Learning Response D: Incorrect.

Learning Response E: Incorrect. Filariasis induces suppression of T_{h2}-type lymphocytes which fail to produce protective IgE and eosinophilia.

---

276. SUBJECT AREA: Core revision
QUESTION: Inflammation is a defensive reaction initiated by infection or tissue injury which *first* causes:

- *A:* Upregulation of adhesion molecules on endothelial cells and leukocytes
- *B:* Chemotaxis
- *C:* IL-8 release
- *D:* Phagocytosis
- *E:* Bacterial killing

☐ Correct Answer: *A*

Learning Response A: Correct. Up-regulation of P-selectin leads to binding to sialyl lewis^x on the PMN and causes rolling along the endothelium. Upregulation of PAF leads to firm binding to the receptor on the PMN and the cell is then subject to chemotactic attraction to pass through the endothelial cells.

Learning Response B: Incorrect. Chemotaxis occurs after anchoring to the endothelial cell.

Learning Response C: Incorrect. The chemotactic IL-8 is released late in inflammation from the endothelial cell.

Learning Response D: Incorrect. Phagocytosis occurs after chemotactic attraction to the target.

Learning Response E: Incorrect. Bacterial killing follows phagocytosis.

277.
SUBJECT AREA: Core revision
QUESTION: Extracellular bacteria are killed by:

- A: Secreting exotoxins
- B: Impeding inflammatory reactions
- C: Phagocytosis and complement
- D: Toxin neutralization
- E: C-reactive protein

☐ Correct Answer: *C*

Learning Response A: Incorrect. Exotoxins are secreted by bacteria and damage the host.

Learning Response B: Incorrect. Inflammatory reactions defend the host and their impedence helps the bacterium.

Learning Response C: Correct. Major killing of extracellular bacteria is through phagocytosis and intracellular killing. Complement aids opsonisation of bacteria to facilitate phagocytosis but may also be responsible for the bactericidal action of fresh serum containing antibody on Gram-negative bacteria.

Learning Response D: Incorrect. Neutralization of toxin helps the host.

Learning Response E: Incorrect. Binding of C-reactive protein to certain bacteria facilitates C1q activation and hence coating with complement which then facilitates various killing processes.

278.
SUBJECT AREA: Core revision
QUESTION: The mucosal surfaces of the body are initially protected by free:

- A: IgG
- B: IgM
- C: IgE
- D: Secretory IgA
- E: IgD

☐ Correct Answer: *D*

Learning Response A: Incorrect. IgG may appear late after initiation of an inflammatory reaction.

Learning Response B: Incorrect. IgM is largely intravascular.

Learning Response C: Incorrect. IgE bound to mast cells acts as a second back-up to infection from the mucosal surface but is not present in the extramucosal space.

Learning Response D: Correct. IgA with secretory piece is dimeric and is the main Ig which prevents adherence of bacteria to the mucosal surface and opsonizes bacteria for adherence to macrophages with Fcα receptors.

Learning Response E: Incorrect. IgD is essentially a lymphocyte surface receptor Ig.

---

279. SUBJECT AREA: Core revision
QUESTION: Bacteria growing within macrophages are killed by:

- *A:* Complement
- *B:* Reactive oxygen and nitrogen intermediates
- *C:* Antibody
- *D:* Cytotoxic T cells
- *E:* Cytokines released from T_{h1} cells

☐ Correct Answer: *B*

Learning Response A: Incorrect. Complement is extracellular and not available to the intracellular bacteria.

Learning Response B: Correct. These mechanisms come into play when the macrophage is activated. Other mechanisms, e.g., peptide defensins and cationic proteins may also contribute to killing.

Learning Response C: Incorrect. Like complement, antibody is extracellular and not available to these bacteria.

Learning Response D: Incorrect. Cytotoxic T cells would kill the macrophage but release the intracellular living bacterium.

Learning Response E: Incorrect. Cytokines from T_{h1} cells do not directly kill but activate the macrophage to facilitate and enhance the killing mechanisms.

280.
SUBJECT AREA: Core revision

QUESTION: Some viruses escape the immune system by antigen *shift*. This involves:

      A: Structural reorganization of existing antigens
      B: Masking of antigen epitopes
      C: Point mutations in single genes
      D: Point mutations in many genes
      E: Interchange of genetic material with other viruses

☐ Correct Answer: *E*

Learning Response A: Incorrect. This may occur with certain parasites such as trypanosomes which change their surface antigens.

Learning Response B: Incorrect.

Learning Response C: Incorrect. Point mutations may reduce the protective response by changing surface antigens but this process of minor antigenic change point mutation is called drift.

Learning Response D: Incorrect. This is a multiple form of drift, if it exists.

Learning Response E: Correct. Antigens which play a major role in establishing protection may be fundamentally altered by interchange of genetic material with an animal viral reservoir.

281.
SUBJECT AREA: Core revision

QUESTION: Protection against worm infestations is particularly associated with an increase in:

      A: IgD
      B: IgE
      C: IgG
      D: IgA
      E: IgM

☐ Correct Answer: *B*

Learning Response A: Incorrect.

Learning Response B: Correct. IgE initiates inflammation which recruits IgG to the site and helps to cause metabolic damage to the worm. Worms are polyclonal stimulators of IgE which will increase competition for the specific IgE by large amounts of irrelevant molecules.

Learning Response C: Incorrect. IgE initiates inflammation which recruits IgG to the site and helps to cause metabolic damage to the worm. Worms are polyclonal stimulators of IgE which will increase competition for the specific IgE by large amounts of irrelevant molecules.

Learning Response D: Incorrect.

Learning Response E: Incorrect.

---

282. SUBJECT AREA: Core revision
QUESTION: Parasites may avoid immune recognition by:

- *A:* Disguising themselves with host protein
- *B:* Variation in their surface antigen
- *C:* Production of non-specific suppression
- *D:* All of the above
- *E:* None of the above

☐ Correct Answer: *D*

Learning Response A: True but not as completely correct as D.

Learning Response B: True but not as completely correct as D.

Learning Response C: True but not as completely correct as D.

Learning Response D: Correct.

Learning Response E: Incorrect.

---

283. SUBJECT AREA: Vaccination
QUESTION: The term variolation refers to:

- *A:* The generation of antibody variable regions
- *B:* The attenuation of virulent organisms
- *C:* Innoculation of scab material into small skin wounds

D: The removal of scab material from an individual with smallpox
E: A type of gene therapy

☐ Correct Answer: *C*

Learning Response A: Incorrect. The variable region on the antibody molecule is encoded by rearranged gene segments; a variable region gene segment and a joining region gene segment in the case of light chains, and additionally a diversity region gene segment in the case of heavy chains. This process of gene rearrangement is referred to as the generation of diversity.

Learning Response B: Incorrect. The objective behind attenuation is to produce a modified organism which mimics the natural behaviour of the original microbe without causing significant disease. In many instances the immunity conferred by live attenuated vaccines is superior to that resulting from killed vaccines. Replication gives a bigger dose and the immune response is produced at the site of the natural infection.

Learning Response C: Correct. Deliberate attempts to ward off infections by inducing a minor form of the disease were common in China in the middle ages. The practice of variolation as a protection against smallpox spread from India, through Turkey and into Western Europe in the 18th century.

Learning Response D: Incorrect. The removal of scab material from an individual recovering from smallpox is not what this term refers to. However, you are very close; try again and you will probably be right!

Learning Response E: Incorrect. The process of variolation was developed several centuries ago. In comparison, gene therapy is a concept only very recently developed.

284. SUBJECT AREA: Core revision
QUESTION: A potential disadvantage of immunological protection using passive transfer of horse globulins is:

A: Serum sickness
B: Irreversible protection
C: Lack of antibody-mediated immune response
D: Type IV hypersensitivity reactions
E: Immunodeficiency

☐ Correct Answer: A

Learning Response A: Correct. Horse globulins containing anti-tetanus and anti-diphtheria toxins have been extensively employed prophylactically, but have the drawback that serum sickness develops in response to foreign proteins, producing vasculitic skin rashes, swollen joints and transient albuminuria due to immune complex-mediated inflammatory reactions.

Learning Response B: Incorrect. The protection only lasts as long as the horse globulins remain in the host, i.e., until catabolism of the protein occurs.

Learning Response C: Incorrect. By far the major component in the γ-globulin fraction is immunoglobulin and thus the basis of the passive transfer is to provide an antibody-mediated immune response.

Learning Response D: Incorrect. However, isolated γ-globulin preparations tend to form small aggregates spontaneously and these can lead to severe anaphylactic reactions when administered intravenously on account of their ability to aggregate platelets and to activate complement, thus generating the C3a and C5a anaphyla-toxins. γ-Globulin preparations are therefore normally given intramuscularly.

Learning Response E: Incorrect. The purpose of passive transfer is to overcome a selective lack of specific antibody.

285. SUBJECT AREA: Passively acquired immunity
QUESTION: The circulation of a two-month-old breast-fed baby will contain maternal:

A: IgA
B: IgD
C: IgE
D: IgG
E: IgM

☐ Correct Answer: D

Learning Response A: Incorrect. There are large amounts of IgA in breast milk, and it is presumed that IgA-producing cells, responding to gut antigens, migrate and colonize breast tissue. However, this secretory IgA is not absorbed by the baby but remains in the intestine to protect the mucosal surfaces.

Learning Response B: Incorrect. Although largely a cell surface-associated immunoglobulin present on virgin B cells, IgD is found in the maternal circulation, albeit in rather small quantities (0–0.4 mg/ml). However, there is no mechanism whereby the maternal IgD can be passed in reasonable amounts to either the fetus or to the newborn.

Learning Response C: Incorrect. IgE is present in the maternal circulation in vanishingly small amounts (17–450 ng/ml) and is not passed to the fetus or newborn.

Learning Response D: Correct. Maternal IgG is transferred across the placenta from the mother to the fetus by a mechanism involving specific Fcγ receptors. IgG is the only immunoglobulin class to cross the placenta. Immunoglobulins in the milk (mostly secretory IgA) will provide enteric protection for the baby but are not absorbed. Thus the maternal immunoglobulin in the circulation of a 2-month-old baby will mostly be placentally-transferred IgG which will provide 'cover' for the first few months of life.

Learning Response E: Incorrect. IgM is neither transferred across the placenta nor present to any great extent in maternal milk.

286. SUBJECT AREA: Passively acquired immunity
QUESTION: An antigen-binding single chain Fv comprises:

- *A:* An entire Ig heavy chain
- *B:* An entire Ig light chain
- *C:* The variable region from an Ig heavy chain
- *D:* The variable region from an Ig light chain
- *E:* The variable region from an Ig heavy and light chain

☐ Correct Answer: *E*

Learning Response A: Incorrect. An interesting recent observation is that immunoglobulins in camels appear to lack light chains. Their antibodies consist of heavy chain dimers which are able to bind to antigen with perfectly respectable affinities.

Learning Response B: Incorrect. Isolated light chains (Bence Jones proteins) are found in the plasma and urine of patients with B-cell malignancies such as multiple myeloma.

Learning Response C: Incorrect. This would be called a V_H domain.

Learning Response D: Incorrect. This would be called a V_L domain.

Learning Response E: Correct. The V region of a heavy chain linked by a flexible spacer molecule to the V region of a light chain is termed a single chain Fv. These are produced using recombinant DNA techniques. They can often bind antigen with reasonable affinity, although being monovalent their functional affinity (avidity) will be the same as their intrinsic affinity.

---

287. SUBJECT AREA: Vaccination

QUESTION: What percentage of children are required to be vaccinated in order to achieve herd immunity to diphtheria:

A: 100%
B: 10%
C: 50%
D: 75%
E: Herd immunity cannot be achieved against diphtheria

☐ Correct Answer: *D*

Learning Response A: Incorrect. The concept of herd immunity relates to the fact that with diseases which spread from one individual to another, depending upon the efficiency of human transmission, not all individuals need to be vaccinated in order to provide overall protection to the community.

Learning Response B: Incorrect. Immunity in just a proportion of the population can help the whole community if it leads to a fall in the number of further cases produced by each infected individual to less than one. However, one would need to vaccinate many more than 10% of a community to achieve this.

Learning Response C: Incorrect. Immunity in just a proportion of the population can help the whole community if it leads to a fall in the number of further cases produced by each infected individual to less than one. However, one would usually need to vaccinate more than 50% of a community to achieve this.

Learning Response D: Correct. Herd immunity can only be achieved in those diseases which depend on human transmission, such as diphtheria. Thus, in the case of tetanus, active immunization is of benefit to the individual but not to the community since it will not eliminate the organism which is found in the feces of domestic animals and persists in soil as highly resistant spores.

Learning Response E: Incorrect. Herd immunity can be achieved against diphtheria, as with other diseases which are spread by human transmission.

---

288. SUBJECT AREA: Vaccination
QUESTION: For vaccination against mycobacterial diseases such as tuberculosis, the most important facet of the immune response to be stimulated is:

A: A high titer of antibody
B: Macrophage-activating cell-mediated immunity
C: Cytotoxic T cells
D: Antibody in the gut lumen
E: Neutrophils

☐ Correct Answer: *B*

Learning Response A: Incorrect. This is more appropriate for organisms such as the poliomyelitis virus where a local nasopharyngeal IgA response at the natural site of infection can be achieved using per oral immunization with live attenuated virus.

Learning Response B: Correct. The objective of vaccination is to provide effective immunity. The particular immune mechanisms that need to be stimulated, and the site of the immune response evoked by vaccination, will differ for different organisms. Mycobacteria are found as intracellular infections within macrophages and therefore stimulating T cells to produce macrophage-activating cytokines such as IFNγ is appropriate in this case.

Learning Response C: Incorrect. Cytotoxic T cells probably play an important role in protection against viruses such as influenza, although some recent evidence points to an accessory role for CD8 T cells in mycobacterial infection.

Learning Response D: Incorrect. Stimulation of an antibody response in the gut lumen would be particularly appropriate for diseases such as cholera where it is desirable to block binding of the bacillus to the intestinal wall in order to prevent subsequent colonization.

Learning Response E: Incorrect. Neutrophils are very important as quick response phagocytes in the immune response but are short lived and are part of the innate immune system; thus they do not show either memory or a high degree of antigen specificity. As the whole basis of vaccination is to prime for a secondary immune response, it is not possible to do this directly for neutrophil-mediated responses.

289. SUBJECT AREA: Killed organisms as vaccines
QUESTION: Which of the following is resistant to lysis by antibody and complement:

- A: Sheep erythrocytes
- B: Neisseria
- C: *Entamoeba histolytica*
- D: $CD8^+$ T cells
- E: $CD4^+$ T cells

☐ Correct Answer: C

Learning Response A: Incorrect. Sheep erythrocytes are readily lysed in the presence of specific antibody and complement, as seen in the hemolytic plaque-forming cell assay used to measure antibody-secreting B lymphocytes.

Learning Response B: Incorrect. The destruction of gonococci by serum which contains specific antibody is dependent upon the formation of the membrane attack complex (MAC). Rare individuals lacking C8 or C9 are susceptible to Neisseria infection.

Learning Response C: Correct. Although *Entamoeba histolytica* is generally resistant to lysis by antibody and complement, it shows greatly increased susceptibility if treated with an otherwise nontoxic protein inhibitor, a feature that could perhaps be exploited in regimes aimed at protection against this organism.

Learning Response D: Incorrect. In fact, the use of antibody to CD8 together with complement can be used to deplete $CD8^+$ T cells from a mixed population of cells.

Learning Response E: Incorrect. In fact, the use of antibody to CD4 together with complement can be used to deplete $CD4^+$ T cells from a mixed population of cells.

290. SUBJECT AREA: Live attenuated organisms as vaccines
QUESTION: Which one of the following diseases has been completely eradicated world-wide:

- A: Poliomyelitis
- B: Smallpox
- C: Tuberculosis
- D: Cowpox
- E: Psittacosis

☐ Correct Answer: *B*

Learning Response A: Incorrect. The continued low incidence of this disease in developed countries is wholly dependent on maintaining the high percentage of individuals which are vaccinated against poliomyelitis.

Learning Response B: Correct. The eradication of smallpox was due to an enormous World Health Organization (WHO)–sponsored effort combining extensive vaccination and selective epidemiologic control methods.

Learning Response C: Incorrect. A major problem worldwide, tuberculosis is the largest cause of death in the world from a single infectious agent. A virulent strain of mycobacterium tuberculosis became attenuated by chance in 1908 when Calmette and Guérin added bile to the culture medium in an attempt to achieve dispersed growth. After 13 years of culture in bile-containing medium, the strain remained attenuated. The same organism, BCG (Bacille Calmette-Guérin) is widely used today for the immunization of tuberculin negative individuals.

Learning Response D: Incorrect. The human equivalent, smallpox, has been completely eradicated but cowpox is still around although this is a nonpathogenic virus in man.

Learning Response E: Incorrect. In this case the chain of infection has been broken by controlling the importation of the parrots which are carriers of this disease.

291. SUBJECT AREA: Live attenuated organisms as vaccines
QUESTION: The first production of live but nonvirulent forms of chicken cholera bacillus was achieved by:

A: Pasteur
B: Salk
C: Jenner
D: Montague
E: Sabin

☐ Correct Answer: *A*

Learning Response A: Correct. A culture of chicken cholera bacillus accidently left on the bench during the warm summer months lost much of its ability to cause disease but could protect birds from the effects of fresh virulent bacillus. Pasteur also obtained similar results for anthrax and rabies.

Learning Response B: Incorrect. The Salk vaccine is killed poliomyelitis virus.

Learning Response C: Incorrect. Edward Jenner showed that prior innoculation with cowpox, which is nonpathogenic in man, protected against subsequent challenge with smallpox. By injecting a harmless form of a disease organism, he had utilized the specificity and memory of the acquired immune response to lay the foundations for modern vaccination (Latin *vacca*, cow).

Learning Response D: Incorrect. Lady Wortley Montague introduced the practice of variolation to Western Europe, a practice that was common in China in the Middle Ages as a means of preventing smallpox.

Learning Response E: Incorrect. The Sabin vaccine is an attenuated poliomyelitis vaccine.

---

292. SUBJECT AREA: Live attenuated organisms as vaccines
QUESTION: BCG is used to protect against:

  A: Tuberculosis
  B: Rabies
  C: Cholera
  D: Influenza
  E: Pertussis

☐ Correct Answer: *A*

Learning Response A: Correct. Bacille Calmette-Guérin (BCG) was developed by Calmette and Guérin by chance in 1908 at the Institut Pasteur in Lille. They added bile to the culture medium in an attempt to achieve dispersed growth of *Mycobacterium tuberculosis,* but it became attenuated and successfully protected vaccinated children against tuberculosis. However, although BCG has been in use for 70 years and is reasonably efficacious and safe in healthy non-T-cell deficient subjects, in some parts of the world it elicits a relatively poor degree of protection against TB and *Mycobacterium leprae*.

Learning Response B: Incorrect. An inactivated viral vaccine can be used prophylactically in high risk groups and post-exposure to contacts in endemic areas.

Learning Response C: Incorrect. An oral vaccine which combines the B subunit of cholera toxin with killed *Vibrio cholerae* stimulates an excellent IgA response in the gut mucosa.

Learning Response D: Incorrect. Both inactivated whole virus and subunit vaccines are available for influenza, but the high degree of variability between strains continues to frustrate attempts to make a universal influenza vaccine. Generally given to the elderly and to high risk groups.

Learning Response E: Incorrect. A triple vaccine (DTP) against diphtheria, tetanus and pertussis is now routinely administered to children in most developed countries.

---

293. SUBJECT AREA: Live attenuated organisms as vaccines
QUESTION: Vaccinia virus vectors cannot be used:

- *A:* In individuals previously immunized with vaccinia used as a smallpox vaccine
- *B:* As part of a vaccine against hepatitis B
- *C:* In B-cell immunodeficient individuals
- *D:* In T-cell immunodeficient individuals
- *E:* To express the IL-2 gene

☐ Correct Answer: *D*

Learning Response A: Incorrect. They can, but there is a chance they will be less effective in this group.

Learning Response B: Incorrect. A wide variety of genes have been expressed in vaccinia virus vectors, including viral envelope proteins such as influenza hemagglutinin, vesicular stomatosis virus glycoprotein, HIV-1 gp120 and herpes simplex virus glycoprotein D. Hepatitis B surface antigen constructs protect chimpanzees against the clinical effects of hepatitis B virus.

Learning Response C: Incorrect. It is probably safe to use vaccinia virus vectors in B-cell immunodeficient individuals.

Learning Response D: Correct. T-cell immunodeficient individuals have difficulty in clearing the virus, although the resistance of nude mice lacking T cells to 10^8 PFUs (plaque-forming units) of recombinant vaccinia expressing the IL-2 gene suggests a way around this problem.

Learning Response E: Incorrect. A wide variety of genes have been expressed in vaccinia virus vectors, including viral envelope proteins such as influenza hemagglutinin, vesicular stomatosis virus glycoprotein, HIV-1 gp120 and herpes simplex virus glycoprotein D. Nude mice largely lacking T cells were resistant to 10^8 PFUs (plaque-forming units) of recombinant vaccinia expressing the IL-2 gene.

294. SUBJECT AREA: Core revision
QUESTION: An attraction of a *Salmonella*-based vaccine expressing antigens from other infectious agents is that:

   A: Immunity is limited to the gut
   B: Only secretory IgA is elicited
   C: It does not invade the mucosal lining of the gut
   D: It provokes both oral and systemic immunity
   E: The organism does not need to be attenuated

☐ Correct Answer: *D*

Learning Response A: Incorrect. The oral route of vaccination may be applicable not only for the establishment of gut mucosal immunity but also for providing systemic protection. *Salmonella typhimurium* not only invades the mucosal lining of the gut but stimulates the production of humoral and secretory antibodies as well as CD4-mediated and CD8-mediated immunity.

Learning Response B: Incorrect. *Salmonella typhimurium* not only invades the mucosal lining of the gut but stimulates the production of humoral and secretory antibodies as well as CD4-mediated and CD8-mediated immunity.

Learning Response C: Incorrect. It does.

Learning Response D: Correct. *Salmonella* infects cells of the mononuclear phagocyte system throughout the body and thereby stimulates the production of cell-mediated immunity in addition to both secretory and systemic antibody production. It can be made to express proteins from *Shigella,* cholera, malarial sporozoites, etc., and has potential as an orally administered vaccine.

Learning Response E: Incorrect. It does, but this is readily achieved.

295. SUBJECT AREA: Core revision
QUESTION: To which one of the following groups would it be acceptable to give a live attenuated viral vaccine:

   A: Children under 8 years of age
   B: Patients treated with steroids
   C: Pregnant mothers
   D: Patients with leukemia
   E: Patients treated with radiotherapy

☐ Correct Answer: *A*

Learning Response A: Correct. Live attenuated organisms can be safely administered to children under 8 years of age so long as they are not immunodeficient. Attenuated vaccines for poliomyelitis (Sabin), measles and rubella have gained general acceptance and are routinely given to babies and infants.

Learning Response B: Incorrect. It is inadvisable to give live vaccines to patients treated with these anti-inflammatory agents since they may be unable to check the growth of these organisms.

Learning Response C: Incorrect. Pregnant mothers should not be given live viral vaccines because the fetus is vulnerable due to a relative lack of T-cell mediated immunity.

Learning Response D: Incorrect. Patients with malignant conditions such as lymphoma and leukemia may well be immunocompromised and therefore should not be given live viral vaccines.

Learning Response E: Incorrect. Patients treated with radiotherapy may well be immunocompromised and therefore should not be given live viral vaccines.

---

296. SUBJECT AREA: Subunit vaccines
QUESTION: Tetanus toxoid is usually given to humans:

      A: Absorbed to aluminum hydroxide
      B: With complete Freund's adjuvant
      C: Without the addition of any other agent
      D: Together with the toxin
      E: Only as a therapeutic agent, not prophylactically

☐ Correct Answer: *A*

Learning Response A: Correct. Bacterial exotoxins can be detoxified by formaldehyde treatment which does not destroy the major immunogenic determinants. The toxoid is generally given after adsorption to aluminum hydroxide, which acts as an adjuvant and produces higher antibody titers.

Learning Response B: Incorrect. Complete Freund's adjuvant is an emulsion of aqueous antigen in mineral oil that contains heat-killed mycobacteria, but its side effects can be rather severe (e.g., granuloma formation) and it is therefore not acceptable for use in humans.

Learning Response C: Incorrect. In the absence of an adjuvant, the immune response to tetanus toxoid is relatively weak.

Learning Response D: Incorrect. If the toxin were administered to humans they would suffer the symptoms of a tetanus infection as it is the toxin which is the disease-causing agent.

Learning Response E: Incorrect. The toxoid is usually used as a prophylactic agent although it can be given to boost antibody titers immediately following natural infection.

---

297. SUBJECT AREA: Subunit vaccines
QUESTION: A small protein subunit used in a vaccine may fail to stimulate T-cell immunity because of:

A: Lack of glycosylation
B: Lack of conformation
C: Lack of carrier determinants
D: HLA-related unresponsiveness
E: Insufficient antigen concentration

☐ Correct Answer: *D*

Learning Response A: Incorrect. The glycosylation of proteins is not thought to directly play a significant role in stimulating T-cell activity, although it may influence the way in which the antigen is processed.

Learning Response B: Incorrect. The T-cell receptor recognizes processed antigen presented by MHC molecules, and therefore the conformation of the protein subunit in a vaccine is probably not of overriding importance.

Learning Response C: Incorrect. The term carrier determinant usually refers to the requirement for a helper T-cell epitope to be linked to a B-cell epitope when wishing to stimulate an antibody response.

Learning Response D: Correct. A major concern about subunit vaccines, especially when just short peptides are used, is the variation in ability to associate with the different polymorphic forms of MHC molecules present in an outbred population.

Learning Response E: Incorrect. Although a threshold of antigen concentration is required to trigger any immune response, this is not a specific feature of subunit vaccines.

298. SUBJECT AREA: Subunit vaccines
QUESTION: Baculovirus vectors can be produced in cell lines derived from which of the following:

   A: Moth
   B: Chicken bursa
   C: Chinese hamster ovary
   D: Tobacco
   E: Green monkey kidney

☐ Correct Answer: *A*

Learning Response A: Correct. Baculovirus vectors in moth cell lines produce large amounts of glycosylated recombinant protein. The baculovirus is a natural infectious agent of insect cells.

Learning Response B: Incorrect. Cells derived from the chicken bursa would usually be B-cell lines, as this organ is the major site of B-lymphocyte development in avian species.

Learning Response C: Incorrect. Chinese hamster ovary (CHO) cells are frequently used in stable expression systems for the production of glycosylated recombinant proteins, but they are not used for the production of baculovirus vectors.

Learning Response D: Incorrect. Whole plants are a good source of large amounts of recombinant proteins, but they take a long time to grow compared to either prokaryotic or eukaryotic cell line expression systems.

Learning Response E: Incorrect. COS cells, derived from green monkey kidney, are often used in transient expression systems for the production of glycosylated recombinant proteins, but they are not used for the production of baculovirus vectors.

299. SUBJECT AREA: Subunit vaccines
QUESTION: Ovine cysticercosis is caused by:

   A: Bacille Calmette-Guérin
   B: Saponin
   C: *S. japonicum*
   D: *Taenia ovis*
   E: Scrapie

☐ Correct Answer: *D*

Learning Response A: Incorrect. Bacille Calmette-Guérin (BCG) is an attenuated *Mycobacterium tuberculosis* used both as a specific vaccine for tuberculosis and as an adjuvant.

Learning Response B: Incorrect. Saponin is not an infectious agent, but rather it is the adjuvant which is used in the vaccine which protects sheep against ovine cysticercosis.

Learning Response C: Incorrect. Glutathione-S-transferase from *S. japonicum* has been used as a fusion partner for the successful isolation of a protective antigen from the early larval oncosphere stage of *Taenia ovis*.

Learning Response D: Correct. These are the larval tapeworms which cause this disease. An extract of the early larval oncosphere stage will immunize completely against reinfection as will a 47–52 kDa antigen from this larval stage.

Learning Response E: Incorrect. Scrapie is a degenerative disease of the central nervous system of sheep, which can spread to cattle to produce bovine spongiform encephalopathy (BSE). A human counterpart of this disease is Creutzfeldt-Jakob disease (CJD). The infectious agents involved in these diseases, termed 'prions', are poorly characterized.

300. SUBJECT AREA: Core revision
QUESTION: An antibody response to a protein vaccine can only be obtained:

A: If the molecule is first linked to a carrier
B: If the molecule maintains discontinuous epitopes
C: If the molecule is glycosylated
D: If disulfide bonds are maintained
E: If the peptide bonds are maintained

☐ Correct Answer: *E*

Learning Response A: Incorrect. Larger molecules will possess their own carrier determinants which provide epitopes for helper T cells. However, subunit vaccines consisting of short peptides must first be coupled to carriers such as tetanus toxoid or mycobacterial heat shock proteins in order to make the peptide immunogenic.

Learning Response B: Incorrect. Although most antibody responses are against discontinuous epitopes, responses can be elicited against continuous (linear) epitopes. However, such epitopes must be accessible on the surface of the native molecule if the antibodies elicited are to be effective in vivo.

Learning Response C: Incorrect. It is not necessary for glycoprotein-derived molecules to be glycosylated in order to elicit strong antibody responses. However, it is important to ensure that the response elicited against the vaccine is directed towards epitopes that are accessible in vivo, e.g., not masked by carbohydrate.

Learning Response D: Incorrect. If the disulfide bonds are reduced the conformation of the protein is likely to be disrupted. However, the molecule will still be immunogenic and this does not cause a problem unless all the native epitopes, including accessible linear sequences, are lost.

Learning Response E: Correct. The peptide bonds hold the amino acids together and if these are not maintained then the vaccine will simply consist of a mixture of amino acids; not much use as a specific vaccine.

---

301. SUBJECT AREA: Subunit vaccines
QUESTION: Short peptides which are virtually universal T-cell epitopes, irrespective of the MHC type of the vaccinee, are called:

- *A:* Histotopes
- *B:* Promiscuous
- *C:* Agretopes
- *D:* Mimotopes
- *E:* Superantigens

☐ Correct Answer: *B*

Learning Response A: Incorrect. The histotope (*histo*compatibility) is that part of the MHC molecule which contacts the T-cell receptor.

Learning Response B: Correct. A major concern regarding peptides as T-cell vaccines is the variation in ability to associate with the different polymorphic variants of MHC molecules present in an outbred population. Some sequences, e.g., residues 378-398 of the malarial circumsporozoite protein, are universal T-cell epitopes recognizable by virtually all individuals so far tested.

Learning Response C: Incorrect. The agretope (Ag recognition) is that part of the T-cell epitope that contacts the MHC molecule.

Learning Response D: Incorrect. A term coined by Geyson to describe short linear peptides which mimic the residues which form an epitope.

Learning Response E: Incorrect. A superantigen is one which reacts with all the T-cells belonging to a particular T-cell receptor V region family, and which therefore stimulates (or deletes) a much larger number of cells than does conventional antigen.

---

302. SUBJECT AREA: Core revision

QUESTION: Idiotypes can be exploited as epitope-specific vaccines if they are:

    A: IgG but not IgM
    B: At least bivalent
    C: First deglycosylated
    D: Only if they are anti-idiotypes
    E: Internal image

☐ Correct Answer: *E*

Learning Response A: Incorrect. The idiotype is associated with the variable region sequence of an antibody (or T-cell receptor) molecule and therefore independent of the constant region which defines class.

Learning Response B: Incorrect. Note, however, that each idiotype will be represented twice on a bivalent antibody molecule (and ten times on pentameric IgM).

Learning Response C: Incorrect. Idiotypes are determined by the amino acid sequence of the antibody variable region. Some are associated with only the V_H, some with only the V_L, whereas others comprise amino acids contributed by both the V_H and V_L domains.

Learning Response D: Incorrect. The term anti-idiotype is really an operational one, in which an antiserum or monoclonal antibody is produced following immunization with an antibody (the 'idiotype'). Jerne's network hypothesis suggests that mutual idiotypic recognition between antibodies forms a network of interactions. In this mutual recognition an antibody is simultaneously both idiotype and anti-idiotype.

Learning Response E: Correct. A problem with using peptides as surrogate antigens is that they are usually unable to mimic discontinuous epitopes. One solution is to produce anti-idiotypes which act as internal images (functional mimics) of the determinant.

303. SUBJECT AREA: Primary innate immunity
QUESTION: Defects in polymorph NADPH oxidase system produce:

- A: Chronic granulomatous disease
- B: Chediak-Higashi disease
- C: Leukocyte adhesion deficiency
- D: Lazy leukocyte syndrome
- E: Streptococcal infection

☐ Correct Answer: *A*

Learning Response A: Correct. There is a failure to make reactive oxygen intermediates and to raise the pH in the phagocytic vacuole which facilitates microbicidal action.

Learning Response B: Incorrect. In this disease lysosomes are deficient in elastase and cathepsin G.

Learning Response C: Incorrect. These patients lack β_2-integrins causing impaired neutrophil chemotaxis.

Learning Response D: Incorrect. There is a defective polymorph response to chemotactic stimuli in this syndrome.

Learning Response E: Incorrect. Organisms which lack catalase to destroy the H_2O_2 generated by their own metabolic processes, and microorganisms which are resistant to oxygen-independent mechanisms are persistent in patients with this deficiency.

304. SUBJECT AREA: Primary innate immunity
QUESTION: Paroxysmal nocturnal hemoglobinuria results from deficiency in:

- A: Myeloperoxidase
- B: Decay accelerating factor (DAF)
- C: Classical pathway C components
- D: C1 inhibitor
- E: C8

☐ Correct Answer: *B*

Learning Response A: Incorrect. Myeloperoxidase deficiency is associated with susceptibility to systemic candidiasis.

Learning Response B: Correct. The spontaneous creation of alternative pathway C3 convertase on the red cell is normally eliminated through membrane bound DAF.

Learning Response C: Incorrect. These deficiencies are associated with the SLE-like syndrome.

Learning Response D: Incorrect. C1 inhibitor deficiency is associated with production of a vasoactive C2 fragment which causes hereditary angioedema.

Learning Response E: Incorrect. These patients are susceptible to *Neisseria* infection.

---

305. SUBJECT AREA: Primary B-cell deficiency
QUESTION: Bruton's congenital agammaglobulinemia results from a mutation in:

    A: Immunoglobulin mRNA splicing
    B: The gene encoding surface 5'-nucleotidase
    C: An HLA gene
    D: The T cell gp39 gene
    E: A tyrosine kinase gene

☐ Correct Answer: *E*

Learning Response A: Incorrect.

Learning Response B: Incorrect. This is associated with common, variable immunodeficiency.

Learning Response C: Incorrect. Note that patients with IgA deficiency, and with common variable immunodeficiency, often have the same HLA haplotypes suggesting a common underlying disorder.

Learning Response D: Incorrect. This is associated with the hyper-IgM syndrome resulting from a failure to signal to the B cell CD40 to bring about Ig class switching.

Learning Response E: Correct.

306. SUBJECT AREA: Primary B-cell deficiency
QUESTION: Di George syndrome results from a defect in:

      A: Purine nucleoside phosphorylase
      B: Sialophorin (CD43)
      C: Thymic development
      D: DNA repair
      E: CD3

☐ Correct Answer: *C*

Learning Response A: Incorrect. This deficiency produces T-cell depression by allowing accumulation of toxic metabolites such as dGTP to which activated T cells are sensitive.

Learning Response B: Incorrect. Deficiency of sialophorin which ligates ICAM-1, leads to the low IgM and poor response to polysaccharides which are a feature of the Wiskott-Aldrich syndrome.

Learning Response C: Correct. Stem cells are unable to differentiate to mature T cells in the absence of the thymic microenvironment.

Learning Response D: Incorrect. This deficiency is associated with chromosome breaks around genes of the Ig supergene family producing associated cellular and Ig deficiency typical of ataxia telangiectasia.

Learning Response E: Incorrect. A mutation in CD3 leads to CMI deficiency through failure to transduce signals through the T-cell receptor.

---

307. SUBJECT AREA: Combined immunodeficiency
QUESTION: A defect in recombinase enzymes leads to:

      A: Reticular dysgenesis
      B: Bare lymphocyte syndrome
      C: Loss of NK cells
      D: Severe combined immunodeficiency (SCID)
      E: Build-up of toxic nucleotide metabolites

☐ Correct Answer: *D*

Learning Response A: Incorrect. There is a loss of lymphoid and myeloid precursors.

Learning Response B: Incorrect. There is a defect in the reaction of a factor with a transacting regulatory protein RF-X which binds to the HLA class II promoter.

Learning Response C: Incorrect. NK cells do not have rearranged receptors.

Learning Response D: Correct. Formation of recombined B- and T-cell receptors for antigen is unobtainable.

Learning Response E: Incorrect. This occurs in adenosine deaminase and purine nucleoside phosphorylase deficiencies.

---

308. SUBJECT AREA: Recognition of immunodeficiencies
QUESTION: Poor skin tests to a range of microbial antigens such as tuberculin and mumps indicate a deficiency of:

- *A:* NK cells
- *B:* T cells
- *C:* B cells
- *D:* Phagocytosis
- *E:* Opsonization

☐ Correct Answer: *B*

Learning Response A: Incorrect. NK cells do not give rise to skin tests.

Learning Response B: Correct. These are delayed type hypersensitivity skin tests which are mediated by T cells.

Learning Response C: Incorrect.

Learning Response D: Incorrect. This has no influence on skin tests.

Learning Response E: Incorrect. Opsonization is unrelated to skin tests but is concerned with facilitating the uptake of particles by phagocytic cells.

---

309. SUBJECT AREA: Secondary immunodeficiency
QUESTION: Secondary immunodeficiency can result from:

- *A:* Malnutrition

B: X-irradiation
C: Viral infection
D: All of the above
E: None of the above

☐ Correct Answer: *E*

Learning Response A: Incorrect. Statement true but not as complete as answer E.

Learning Response B: Incorrect. Statement true but not as complete as answer E.

Learning Response C: Incorrect. Statement true but not as complete as answer E.

Learning Response D: Incorrect.

Learning Response E: Correct.

---

310. SUBJECT AREA: AIDS
QUESTION: Human acquired immunodeficiency syndrome is initiated by infection with:

A: Visna virus
B: Cytomegalovirus
C: HTLV-1
D: Pneumocystis carinii
E: HIV-1/2

☐ Correct Answer: *E*

Learning Response A: Incorrect. The visna virus is a slow retrovirus like HIV but which gives rise to CNS and lung lesions in sheep.

Learning Response B: Incorrect. Cytomegalovirus infections are common in immunologically compromised patients with AIDS.

Learning Response C: Incorrect. True that HTLV-1 is a retrovirus like HIV, but gives rise instead to human leukemia.

Learning Response D: Incorrect. This is an opportunist infection which frequently infects AIDS patients.

Learning Response E: Correct.

311. SUBJECT AREA: AIDS
QUESTION: HIV binds to:

> A: CD4
> B: CD8
> C: NFκB
> D: Reverse transcriptase
> E: TNF receptors

☐ Correct Answer: *A*

Learning Response A: Correct. The HIV envelope protein gp120 binds to CD4. This targets the virus to this T-cell subset.

Learning Response B: Incorrect.

Learning Response C: Incorrect. This is an intracellular transcription factor whose activation upregulates HIV replication.

Learning Response D: Incorrect. This is the viral enzyme which transcribes viral RNA into DNA.

Learning Response E: Incorrect. TNF presumably reacting with surface TNF surface receptors upregulates HIV replication.

312. SUBJECT AREA: AIDS
QUESTION: The main site of sequestration of HIV in lymphoid tissue is:

> A: Subcapsular sinuses
> B: Medullary cords
> C: Secondary follicles
> D: Paracortical area
> E: Medullary sinuses

☐ Correct Answer: *C*

Learning Response A: Incorrect.

Learning Response B: Incorrect.

Learning Response C: Correct. This leads to ultimate destruction of the secondary follicles that are concerned with secondary B-cell responses.

Learning Response D: Incorrect.

Learning Response E: Incorrect.

---

313. SUBJECT AREA: AIDS
QUESTION: HIV may cause the lesions of AIDS by:

    A: Increasing susceptibility to apoptosis
    B: A direct cytopathic effect on T cells
    C: Causing defective antigen presentation
    D: All of the above
    E: None of the above

☐ Correct Answer: *D*

Learning Response A: Incorrect. The answer is possible but answer D is more complete.

Learning Response B: Incorrect. The answer is possible but answer D is more complete.

Learning Response C: Incorrect. The answer is possible but answer D is more complete.

Learning Response D: Correct.

Learning Response E: Incorrect.

---

314. SUBJECT AREA: AIDS
QUESTION: Which of the following is *not helpful* in the diagnosis of AIDS:

    A: CD4 numbers
    B: CD8 numbers
    C: Skin tests to bacterial antigens
    D: Lymph node biopsy
    E: Serum p24 antigen

☐ Correct Answer: *B*

Learning Response A: Incorrect. CD4 numbers decrease drastically as AIDS progresses clinically.

Learning Response B: Correct. CD8 numbers are largely unaffected. It is the CD4:CD8 ratio that falls dramatically.

Learning Response C: Incorrect. Many delayed hypersensitivity tests to bacterial antigens which depend on T-cell activity, are depressed in AIDS.

Learning Response D: Incorrect. There are drastic changes in germinal centers.

Learning Response E: Incorrect. p24 rises significantly during progression of clinical AIDS.

---

315. SUBJECT AREA: AIDS
QUESTION: Which of the following HIV antigens provides a potential target for neutralizing antibody:

   A: p24
   B: gp120
   C: Reverse transcriptase
   D: Protease
   E: None of the above

☐ Correct Answer: *B*

Learning Response A: Incorrect. This is an intraviral antigen.

Learning Response B: Correct. gp120 is an envelope protein which binds to CD4 on the T cell. Antibodies to the GPGR epitope on the V3 loop of gp120 are particularly effective as neutralizing agents.

Learning Response C: Incorrect. The reverse transcriptase is intraviral and not available to neutralizing antibody.

Learning Response D: Incorrect. Protease is intraviral and splits gp160 into the gp120 and gp41 which is involved in membrane fusion. The protease is not available to neutralizing antibody.

Learning Response E: Incorrect.

316. SUBJECT AREA: AIDS
QUESTION: AZT:

      A: Prevents viral/cell fusion
      B: Blocks gp120/CD4 interaction
      C: Inhibits the HIV protease
      D: Inhibits a carbohydrate trimming enzyme
      E: Inhibits reverse transcriptase

☐ Correct Answer: *E*

Learning Response A: Incorrect.

Learning Response B: Incorrect.

Learning Response C: Incorrect. Some peptide drugs are targetting this protease which is essential for splitting gp160 into the 120 and 41 components.

Learning Response D: Incorrect. Some drugs are targetting this enzyme.

Learning Response E: Correct. Conversion of the viral RNA into DNA is necessary for viral replication.

---

317. SUBJECT AREA: Core revision
QUESTION: Primary immunodeficiency producing susceptibility to infection by viruses and molds is due to:

      A: B-cell deficiency
      B: T-cell deficiency
      C: Phagocyte deficiency
      D: Complement deficiency
      E: None of the above

☐ Correct Answer: *B*

Learning Response A: Incorrect. B-cell deficiency produces susceptibility to infection by pyogenic bacteria which are extracellular.

Learning Response B: Correct. Production of cytokines and of cytotoxic T cells are important in the protective response.

Learning Response C: Incorrect. Phagocyte deficiency predisposes to pyogenic infection.

Learning Response D: Incorrect. Complement deficiency predisposes to pyogenic bacterial infection.

Learning Response E: Incorrect. T-cell deficiency is important.

---

318. SUBJECT AREA: Core revision
QUESTION: Chronic granulomatous disease results from mutations in:

- *A:* β2-integrins
- *B:* Decay accelerating factor (DAF)
- *C:* C1 inhibitor
- *D:* Early classical complement components
- *E:* NADPH oxidase of phagocytic cells

☐ Correct Answer: *E*

Learning Response A: Incorrect. Deficiency of the β2-integrins leads to leukocyte adhesion deficiency.

Learning Response B: Incorrect. DAF deficiency underlies paroxysmal nocturnal hemaglobinuria.

Learning Response C: Incorrect. C1 inhibitor deficiency leads to hereditary angioedema.

Learning Response D: Incorrect. This deficiency is associated with SLE-like syndromes.

Learning Response E: Correct. Lack of the oxidase prevents generation of reactive oxygen intermediates and hence defect in bacterial killing.

---

319. SUBJECT AREA: Core revision
QUESTION: Deletions in the T-cell gp39 gene produce:

- *A:* The hyper-IgM syndrome
- *B:* Congenital X-linked agammaglobulinemia
- *C:* IgA deficiency
- *D:* Common variable immunodeficiency
- *E:* Deficiency in cell-mediated immunity

☐ Correct Answer: *A*

Learning Response A: Correct. Lack of gp39 prevents signalling to the B cell CD40 to bring about Ig class-switching away from IgM.

Learning Response B: Incorrect. This condition involves a defect of the pre-B-cell stage through mutations in a novel tyrosine kinase gene.

Learning Response C: Incorrect. The failure of IgA bearing lymphocytes to become plasma cells is often associated with antibodies to IgA.

Learning Response D: Incorrect. B cells with surface Ig are either missing or present in subnormal numbers. Some T cells have low surface 5'-nucleotidase and lack the non-specific esterase spot. 30% of patients have poor responses to PHA and a small proportion have suppressor T cells active against B cells.

Learning Response E: Incorrect. The deficiency is in T-helper cell activity for B cells.

---

320. SUBJECT AREA: Core revision
QUESTION: Di George syndrome results from:

        A: Defective DNA repair mechanisms
        B: Defect in combinatorial joining of receptor V, D and J genes
        C: Failure of thymic development
        D: Lack of sialophorin
        E: Adenosine deaminase deficiency

☐ Correct Answer: *C*

Learning Response A: Incorrect. This is a characteristic of patients with ataxia telangiectasia.

Learning Response B: Incorrect. This characterizes patients with severe combined immunodeficiency.

Learning Response C: Correct. Without a thymus the T-cell stem cells cannot differentiate.

Learning Response D: Incorrect. Lack of sialophorin, a ligand for ICAM-1, is characteristic of the Wiskott-Aldrich syndrome.

Learning Response E: Incorrect. This affects both B and particularly T cells by accumulation of toxic metabolites of the purine dATP and leads to combined immunodeficiency.

---

321. SUBJECT AREA: Core revision
QUESTION: Which of the following *have not* provided examples of secondary immunodeficiency:

    A: Viral infection
    B: Lymphoproliferative disorders
    C: Cytotoxic drugs
    D: High fat diet
    E: Low iron diet

☐ Correct Answer: *D*

Learning Response A: Incorrect.

Learning Response B: Incorrect.

Learning Response C: Incorrect.

Learning Response D: Correct.

Learning Response E: Incorrect.

---

322. SUBJECT AREA: Core revision
QUESTION: AIDS is associated with:

    A: CD4 T-cell depletion
    B: CD8 T-cell depletion
    C: Polymorph depletion
    D: Pneumococcal infection
    E: Low immunoglobulin levels

☐ Correct Answer: *A*

Learning Response A: Correct. HIV envelope gp120 binds to CD4 and ultimately leads to depletion of this subset.

Learning Response B: Incorrect. CD8 cells are either unaffected or slightly increased so that the CD4:CD8 ratio drops.

Learning Response C: Incorrect. Polymorphs are not affected but macrophages and dendritic cells can be.

Learning Response D: Incorrect. Failure in cell-mediated defenses predisposes to infection with opportunist organisms such as *Pneumocystis carinii* and cytomegalovirus.

Learning Response E: Incorrect. Patients have hypergammaglobulinemia and large numbers of B cells which spontaneously secrete Ig in culture, suggesting polyclonal stimulation.

---

323. SUBJECT AREA: Core revision
QUESTION: Which of the following hypersensitivity states is mediated by T cells:

A: Type I
B: Type II
C: Type III
D: Type IV
E: Type V

☐ Correct Answer: *D*

Learning Response A: Incorrect. Type I is anaphylactic hypersensitivity which depends upon the reaction of antigen with specific IgE antibodies bound through their Fc to the mast cell. Cross-linking of the IgE receptors leads to release from the granules of mediators including histamine, leukotrienes and platelet activating factor, plus eosinophil and neutrophil chemotactic factors and IL-3, -4, -5 and GM-CSF.

Learning Response B: Incorrect. Type II is antibody-dependent cytotoxic hypersensitivity which involves the death of cells bearing antibody attached to a surface antigen. The cells may be taken up by phagocytic cells to which they adhere through their coating of IgG or C3b, or lysed by complement. Cells bearing IgG may also be killed by ADCC.

Learning Response C: Incorrect. Type III is immune complex-mediated hypersensitivity from the effects of antigen-antibody complexes through activation of complement and attraction of polymorphonuclear leukocytes which release tissue-damaging mediators on contact with the complex, and through aggregation of platelets to cause microthrombi and vasoactive amine release.

Learning Response D: Correct. Type IV is cell-mediated or delayed-type hypersensitivity based upon the interaction of antigen with primed T cells and represents tissue damage resulting from inappropriate CMI reactions.

Learning Response E: Incorrect. Type V is stimulatory hypersensitivity in which antibody reacts with a key surface component such as a hormone receptor and 'switches on' the cell.

---

324. SUBJECT AREA: Core revision
QUESTION: Type IV hypersensitivity is often referred to as:

- *A:* Immediate
- *B:* Delayed
- *C:* Anaphylactic
- *D:* Anergic
- *E:* Allotypic

☐ Correct Answer: *B*

Learning Response A: Incorrect. Types I, II, III and V hypersensitivity reactions depend on the interaction of antigen with humoral antibody and tend to be called 'immediate' type reactions, although some are more immediate than others.

Learning Response B: Correct. Type IV hypersensitivity involves T-cell recognition and because of the longer time course of the reaction to intradermal antigen, this is sometimes referred to as delayed-type hypersensitivity.

Learning Response C: Incorrect. The term anaphylactic is nowadays used to refer to type I (IgE-mediated) hypersensitivity although historically it refers to the development of any type of sensitivity to relatively harmless substances. The term anaphylaxis was used in contrast to the term prophylaxis.

Learning Response D: Incorrect. Anergy refers to the potentially reversible specific immunological tolerance in which the lymphocyte becomes functionally nonresponsive. Certainly not hypersensitivity!

Learning Response E: Incorrect. Allotype refers to phenotypic variation encoded by alleles—alternative forms of a gene at a single locus. Because the allelic variant of an antigen is not present in all individuals, the variant may be immunogenic in members of the same species which have a different version of the allele.

325. SUBJECT AREA: Type I hypersensitivity
QUESTION: Passive cutaneous anaphylaxis (PCA) involves the transfer of:

    A: T cells
    B: IgA
    C: IgY
    D: IgE
    E: C5a

☐ Correct Answer: *D*

Learning Response A: Incorrect. The transfer of sensitized T cells provides the recipient with active cell-mediated immunity.

Learning Response B: Incorrect. The transfer of antibody of any isotype from one animal to another is referred to as passive transfer.

Learning Response C: Incorrect. There is no such class of antibody in mammals, although a particular class of avian immunoglobulin is sometimes termed IgY and is most equivalent to mammalian IgG.

Learning Response D: Correct. Passive transfer of anaphylactic sensitivity can be observed locally in the skin using Ovary's passive cutaneous anaphylaxis (PCA) technique. High dilutions of guinea pig serum containing anaphylactic IgE antibodies may be injected into the skin of a normal animal and, following intravenous injection of antigen with a dye such as Evan's blue, the anaphylactic reaction in the skin will lead to the release of vasoactive amines and hence a local 'blueing.'

Learning Response E: Incorrect. However, like C3a and C4a, this complement component acts as an anaphylatoxin; a substance capable of directly triggering mast cell degranulation.

326. SUBJECT AREA: Core revision
QUESTION: Anaphylaxis can be trigerred by cross-linking of IgE receptors on:

    A: Macrophages
    B: Mast cells
    C: B cells
    D: Eosinophils
    E: Neutrophils

☐ Correct Answer: *B*

Learning Response A: Incorrect. CD23 (FcεRII), the low affinity IgE receptor, is present on activated macrophages. However, cross-linking does not result in anaphylaxis.

Learning Response B: Correct. Cross-linking of IgE antibodies bound to the high affinity IgE receptor (FcεRI) on mast cells by a divalent hapten will trigger mediator release; trimers are more effective and tetramers even more so. Degranulation is also induced when the IgE is cross-linked with anti-IgE but univalent (Fab) anti-IgE is inactive. That the critical event is the cross-linking of the receptors themselves is clearly shown by the ability of antibodies reacting directly with the receptor to trigger the mast cell.

Learning Response C: Incorrect. CD23 (FcεRII), the low affinity IgE receptor, is present on a subset of B cells. However, cross-linking does not result in anaphylaxis.

Learning Response D: Incorrect. CD23 (FcεRII), the low affinity IgE receptor, is present on eosinophils. However, cross-linking does not result in anaphylaxis.

Learning Response E: Incorrect. Neutrophils do not possess either the low affinity (FcεRII, CD23) nor the high affinity (FcεRI) IgE receptor.

327. SUBJECT AREA: Type I hypersensitivity
QUESTION: Which one of the following mast cell products is not preformed and therefore has to be newly synthesized:

A: Histamine
B: Prostaglandin D_2
C: Heparin
D: Platelet-activating factor (PAF)
E: Eosinophil chemotactic factor (ECF)

☐ Correct Answer: *B*

Learning Response A: Incorrect. Histamine is preformed and stored in mast cell granules. Upon release it causes vasodilation, increased capillary permeability, chemokinesis and brochoconstriction.

Learning Response B: Correct. Prostaglandins and thromboxanes are newly synthesized by the mast cell using the cyclo-oxygenase pathway. The leukotrienes

B_4, C_4 and D_4 (slow reacting substance of anaphylaxis, SRS-A) are also newly synthesized by the mast cell, in this instance using the lipoxygenase pathway.

Learning Response C: Incorrect. Heparin is preformed and stored in mast cell granules.

Learning Response D: Incorrect. Platelet-activating factor (PAF) is preformed and stored in mast cell granules.

Learning Response E: Incorrect. Eosinophil chemotactic factor (ECF) is preformed and stored in mast cell granules.

328. SUBJECT AREA: Type I hypersensitivity
QUESTION: Lol pI-V are allergens cloned from:

  A: Rye grass pollen
  B: House dust mite
  C: House dust mite feces
  D: Animal danders
  E: *Myrmecia pilosula*

☐ Correct Answer: *A*

Learning Response A: Correct. Nearly 10% of the population suffer to a greater or lesser degree from allergies involving localized IgE-mediated anaphylactic reactions to extrinsic allergens. An increasing number of these allergens have now been cloned including Der p1 from house dust mites and Lol pI-V from rye grass pollen.

Learning Response B: Incorrect. The Der p1 allergen has been cloned from the house dust mite *Dermatophagoides pteryonyssinus* and shown to provoke asthma and eczema.

Learning Response C: Incorrect. The house dust mite is a major cause of allergic disease and its fecal pellets are the main source of the allergen.

Learning Response D: Incorrect. Animal danders can be responsible for provoking either asthma or eczema.

Learning Response E: Incorrect. *Myrmecia pilosula* is the Australian jumper ant, an insect from which an allergen present in venom was identified using IgE screening of a cDNA library.

329. SUBJECT AREA: Type I hypersensitivity
QUESTION: The Praunitz-Kustner test can be blocked using:

    A: Histamine
    B: An IgA myeloma
    C: A myeloma protein of mixed antibody class
    D: Sodium cromoglycate
    E: Interleukin-5

☐ Correct Answer: *D*

Learning Response A: Incorrect. Histamine is a vasoactive amine which will be released from mast cells during the Praunitz-Kustner test and is responsible for many of the symptoms of type I hypersensitivity.

Learning Response B: Incorrect. This passive sensitization of human skin can be blocked most effectively by prior injection of a myeloma of IgE rather than of any other class.

Learning Response C: Incorrect. This is a contradiction because a myeloma, being monoclonal, can only be of a single light chain class.

Learning Response D: Correct. Sodium cromoglycate is a mast cell stabilizer which makes the cell resistant to triggering. It is thus able to block the Praunitz-Kustner test in which patient's serum is used to passively sensitize the skin of normal humans or monkeys before challenge with antigen (allergen) into the prepared site.

Learning Response E: Incorrect. IL-5 primes eosinophils for enhanced locomotor attraction towards mast cells.

330. SUBJECT AREA: Type II hypersensitivity
QUESTION: A major unresolved question concerning ADCC is whether:

    A: Antibody is involved
    B: It can be carried out by NK cells
    C: It leads to cell death
    D: It is complement-dependent
    E: It occurs in vivo

☐ Correct Answer: *E*

Learning Response A: Incorrect. ADCC is antibody-dependent cell-mediated cytotoxicity and therefore, by definition, involves antibody. Specific IgG antibodies target the cytotoxicity by effector cells which have bound the antibody via cell surface Fcγ receptors.

Learning Response B: Incorrect. ADCC can be carried out by a number of Fcγ receptor-bearing cell types including monocytes, macrophages, neutrophils and NK cells.

Learning Response C: Incorrect. ADCC is antibody-dependent cell-mediated cytotoxicity and therefore, by definition, leads to the death of the target cell.

Learning Response D: Incorrect. ADCC is dependent on antibody but not on complement although bound C3 can enhance the reaction if the effector cells bear C3b receptors.

Learning Response E: Correct. This phenomenon is well established in vitro but it is still unclear if it has a role in vivo.

---

331. SUBJECT AREA: Core revision
QUESTION: Rhesus hemolytic disease of the newborn involves:

A: IgE
B: Antibody to cell surfaces
C: Soluble immune complexes
D: Cytokine release from T cells
E: Stimulatory antibodies

☐ Correct Answer: *B*

Learning Response A: Incorrect. Rhesus incompatibility is not a type I (IgE-mediated) hypersensitivity reaction.

Learning Response B: Correct. Rhesus incompatibility between mother and fetus leads to a type II hypersensitivity reaction due to IgG antibodies to the fetal RhD crossing the placenta.

Learning Response C: Incorrect. Rhesus incompatibility does not lead to type III (immune complex-mediated) hypersensitivity reaction.

Learning Response D: Incorrect. Rhesus incompatibility does not lead to type IV T-cell–mediated (delayed-type) hypersensitivity reaction.

Learning Response E: Incorrect. Rhesus incompatibility does not lead to type V hypersensitivity reaction involving stimulatory antibodies.

---

332. SUBJECT AREA: Type II hypersensitivity
QUESTION: *Mycoplasma pneumoniae* infection can lead to:

        A: Hashimoto's thyroiditis
        B: Agranulocytosis
        C: Cold hemagglutinin disease
        D: Thrombocytopenic purpura
        E: Neonatal alloimmune thrombocytopenia

☐ Correct Answer: *C*

Learning Response A: Incorrect. In Hashimoto's thyroiditis, sera contain antibodies which in the presence of complement are directly cytotoxic for isolated human thyroid cells in culture. However, evidence from animal models and the recovery of thyroid-specific T cells from diseased glands suggests an important role for type IV hypersensitivity.

Learning Response B: Incorrect. However, a type II hypersensitivity leading to agranulocytosis is associated with taking the drugs amidopyrine and quinidine.

Learning Response C: Correct. Patients with cold hemagglutinin disease have monoclonal anti-blood group I, leading to an autoimmune hemolytic anemia. The mechanism behind this is unclear but it does not appear to be due to cross-reaction between a mycoplasma antigen and blood group I. It may be that the lipid-rich mycoplasma acts as an adjuvant which overcomes tolerance to the self blood group I antigen.

Learning Response D: Incorrect. Thrombocytopenic purpura may be produced by the sedative Sedormid. The drug appears to form an antigen complex with platelets and evokes the production of antibodies which are cytotoxic for the cell-drug complex in a complement-dependent manner.

Learning Response E: Incorrect. Transplacental transfer of maternal antibodies can result in neonatal alloimmune thrombocytopenia. The fall in platelet numbers is greatly ameliorated by high dose intravenous injections of pooled human IgG, the mechanism being thought to involved anti-idiotype networks.

333. SUBJECT AREA: Type III hypersensitivity
QUESTION: The term *reactive lysis* usually refers to a sequence of events involving:

- *A:* NK cells
- *B:* Cytotoxic T lymphocytes (CTL)
- *C:* Antibody-dependent cell-mediated cytotoxicity (ADCC)
- *D:* Killer (K) cells
- *E:* Complement

☐ Correct Answer: *E*

Learning Response A: Incorrect. NK cells can mediate killing of a range of target cells but this is not referred to as reactive lysis.

Learning Response B: Incorrect. CTL can specifically kill target cells bearing a peptide-MHC complex recognized by the T-cell receptor. They do this using a pore-forming molecule called perforin but this process is not referred to as reactive lysis.

Learning Response C: Incorrect. ADCC is a cytotoxicity mechanism as the name suggests, but it is not referred to as reactive lysis.

Learning Response D: Incorrect. K cells, a population which largely overlaps with NK cells, are able to destroy target cells using antibody-dependent cell-mediated cytotoxicity (ADCC).

Learning Response E: Correct. Following type III hypersensitivity reactions, activated C5b, 6, 7 becomes adventitiously attached to the surface of nearby cells and binds C8, 9 to cause innocent cell death.

334. SUBJECT AREA: Core revision
QUESTION: The Arthus reaction is characterized by an intense infiltration by:

- *A:* Mast cells
- *B:* Polymorphs
- *C:* Eosinophils
- *D:* Macrophages
- *E:* Langerhans' cells

☐ Correct Answer: *B*

Learning Response A: Incorrect. Mast cells are involved in type I anaphylactic hypersensitivity reactions which depend upon the reaction of antigen with specific IgE antibody bound through its Fc to the mast cell.

Learning Response B: Correct. The Arthus reaction is a type III immune complex-mediated hypersensitivity in the skin characterized by polymorph infiltration, edema and erythema maximal at 3–8 hours.

Learning Response C: Incorrect. Serious prolongation of the response to allergen in type I hypersensitivity reactions is caused by T cells of the T_{h2}-type which recruit tissue-damaging eosinophils through the release of IL-5.

Learning Response D: Incorrect. In type IV reactions a number of soluble cytokines including IFNγ are released which activate macrophages and account for the events which occur in a typical delayed-type hypersensitivity response such as the Mantoux reaction to tuberculin.

Learning Response E: Incorrect. Langerhans' cells are MHC class II$^+$ antigen-presenting dendritic cells found in the skin, but are not directly involved in the Arthus reaction which is a type III hypersensitivity reaction in the skin.

335. SUBJECT AREA: Type III hypersensitivity
QUESTION: Maple bark stripper's disease is a hypersensitivity largely affecting the:

A: Skin
B: Kidneys
C: Nervous system
D: Lung
E: Platelets

☐ Correct Answer: *D*

Learning Response A: Incorrect. Many hypersensitivity reactions manifest themselves in the skin, e.g., atopic eczema (type I) and contact dermatitis (type IV), but maple bark stripper's disease does not primarily affect the skin.

Learning Response B: Incorrect. Immune-complex glomerulonephritis is a type III hypersensitivity associated with the autoimmune disease systemic lupus erythematosus (SLE) or with infections by streptococci, malaria and other parasites.

Learning Response C: Incorrect. The choroid plexus is a major filtration site and therefore in type III hypersensitivity is often the site of immune-complex deposition. This may account for the frequency of central nervous system disorders in systemic lupus.

Learning Response D: Correct. Maple bark stripper's disease is a type III extrinsic allergic alveolitis due to continual inhalation of Cryptostroma spores which produce high antibody levels. Similar reactions occur in farmer's lung (thermophilic actinomycetes in mouldy hay), pigeon-fancier's disease (serum protein in dried feces), cheese washer's disease (*Penicillium casei* spores) and furrier's lung (fox fur proteins).

Learning Response E: Incorrect. Type II hypersensitivity reactions are responsible for neonatal alloimmune thrombocytopenia and drug-associated thrombocytopenia purpura.

336. SUBJECT AREA: Type III hypersensitivity
QUESTION: Dead *Wuchereria bancrofti* can cause:

A: Elephantiasis
B: Erythema nodosum leprosum
C: Serum sickness
D: Pigeon fancier's disease
E: Farmer's lung

☐ Correct Answer: *A*

Learning Response A: Correct. Dead filarial worm parasites in lymphatic vessels initiate an inflammatory reaction thought to be responsible for obstruction of the flow of lymph.

Learning Response B: Incorrect. Erythema nodosum leprosum is an immune complex-mediated reaction in the skin of Dapsone-treated lepromatous leprosy patients.

Learning Response C: Incorrect. Serum sickness is caused by the injection of relatively large doses of foreign serum (e.g., horse anti-diphtheria) which used to be employed for various therapeutic purposes. This type III hypersensitivity often arose several days following the injection and is thought to be due to the deposition of soluble antigen-antibody complexes produced in antigen excess.

Learning Response D: Incorrect. Pigeon fancier's disease is a type III hypersensitivity probably caused by serum proteins present in dust from dried feces.

Learning Response E: Incorrect. Farmer's lung is a type III hypersensitivity caused by thermophilic actinomycetes in dust from mouldy hay. It occurs within 6–8 hours of exposure, and patients experience severe respiratory difficulties.

---

337. SUBJECT AREA: Core revision
QUESTION: The injection of tuberculin into the skin of a sensitized individual elicits a(n):

  A: Immune complex glomerulonephritis
  B: Jarisch-Herxheimer reaction
  C: Isohemagglutinins
  D: Jones-Mote sensitivity
  E: Mantoux reaction

☐ Correct Answer: *E*

Learning Response A: Incorrect. Immune complex glomerulonephritis is a type III hypersensitivity associated with the autoimmune disease systemic lupus erythematosus (SLE) or with infections by streptococci, malaria and other parasites.

Learning Response B: Incorrect. The Jarisch-Herxheimer reaction is a type III hypersensitivity in syphilitics being treated with penicillin.

Learning Response C: Incorrect. Isohemagglutinins are antibodies to blood group A or B antigens, usually of the IgM isotype, and probably natural antibodies against carbohydrates on gut microflora. They cause a type II hypersensitivity.

Learning Response D: Incorrect. Jones-Mote sensitivity is similar to a Mantoux reaction and is a delayed-type hypersensitivity (DTH) to soluble proteins, although it is of shorter duration than the Mantoux reaction and is associated with a cutaneous basophil hypersensitivity.

Learning Response E: Correct. A type IV delayed-type hypersensitivity characterized by erythema and induration which appears only after several hours and reaches a maximum at 24–48 hours, by which time the predominant cell types are lymphocytes and monocytes/macrophages.

---

338. SUBJECT AREA: Type IV hypersensitivity
QUESTION: Which type of hypersensitivity cannot be transferred with serum antibody:

A: Type I
B: Type II
C: Type III
D: Type IV
E: Type V

☐ Correct Answer: *D*

Learning Response A: Incorrect. Type I hypersensitivity is caused by IgE antibodies which are transferred in the passive cutaneous anaphylaxis (PCA) technique.

Learning Response B: Incorrect. Type II hypersensitivity is caused by antibodies to cell surfaces. In rhesus incompatibility it is maternal antibodies of the IgG class which cross the placenta and cause hemolytic disease of the newborn.

Learning Response C: Incorrect. Type III hypersensitivity is caused by antibody-containing immune complexes, which leads to undesirable complement activation and other immunopathological events.

Learning Response D: Correct. Unlike the other types of hypersensitivity (I, II, III and V), type IV delayed-type reactivity cannot be transferred from a sensitized to a nonsensitized individual with serum antibody. Lymphoid cells, in particular T lymphocytes, are required.

Learning Response E: Incorrect. Type V is a stimulatory hypersensitivity caused by, for example, autoantibodies to hormone receptors which mimic the effect of the hormone. In neonatal thyrotoxicosis it is transplacental transfer of the maternal stimulatory antibody that causes a transient hyperthyroidism in the neonate.

339. SUBJECT AREA: Core revision
QUESTION: The major effector molecules involved in type IV hypersensitivity reactions are:

A: Antibodies
B: Complement components
C: Cytokines
D: Prostaglandins
E: 5-hydroxytryptamine (5-HT)

☐ Correct Answer: *C*

Learning Response A: Incorrect. Antibodies are the main primary effector molecules in the other types of hypersensitivity reactions, but not in type IV hypersensitivity. Note that the tissue damage itself is usually caused by molecules other than the antibody, e.g., histamine in type I hypersensitivity, phagocytes in type II hypersensitivity.

Learning Response B: Incorrect. Complement components often play a key role in type II and type III hypersensitivity reactions.

Learning Response C: Correct. Type IV hypersensitivity is based upon the interaction of antigen with primed T cells which then release cytokines which mediate the events which occur in this type of hypersensitivity.

Learning Response D: Incorrect. In type I hypersensitivity the mast cell releases a number of mediators, some are preformed and released from granules (e.g., histamine, heparin, platelet-activating factor), whereas others, including prostaglandin D_2 and the leukotrienes, are newly synthesized.

Learning Response E: Incorrect. 5-hydroxytryptamine (5-HT) is released from platelets, e.g., in type III reactions.

340. SUBJECT AREA: Type IV hypersensitivity
QUESTION: Chronic granuloma represents an attempt by the body to:

    A: Wall off a site of chronic infection
    B: Make a site of chronic infection accessible
    C: Digest antibody-antigen complexes
    D: Initiate an immune response
    E: Change from a Th_1 to a Th_2 type of response.

☐ Correct Answer: *A*

Learning Response A: Correct. A granuloma is a tissue nodule containing proliferating lymphocytes, fibroblasts, and giant cells/epithelioid cells (both derived from activated macrophages), which forms due to inflammation in response to chronic infection or persistence of antigen in the tissues.

Learning Response B: Incorrect. A granuloma would not make a site of chronic infection accessible.

Learning Response C: Incorrect. Chronic granuloma can arise from the persistence of undigestible material such as certain immune complexes or inorganic material such as talc within macrophages.

Learning Response D: Incorrect. A chronic granuloma is an ongoing immune response, not a newly initiated one.

Learning Response E: Incorrect. Within a granuloma, Th_1 cells attract and activate macrophages. Th_2 cells attract and activate eosinophils.

341. SUBJECT AREA: Type V hypersensitivity
QUESTION: In thyroid autoimmunity, an antibody causing type V hypersensitivity may be present and is directed against:

A: Thyroglobulin
B: Thyroid peroxidase
C: Thyroid stimulating hormone (TSH) receptor
D: Acetylcholine receptor
E: Thyroxine

☐ Correct Answer: *C*

Learning Response A: Incorrect. Many patients with thyroid autoimmunity have antibodies against thyroglobulin, but their role in pathogenesis (if any) is unknown and they do not cause a type V hypersensitivity.

Learning Response B: Incorrect. Many patients with thyroid autoimmunity have antibodies against thyroid peroxidase (TPO), which could cause type II hypersensitivity complement-mediated tissue damage.

Learning Response C: Correct. The thyroid-stimulatory autoantibodies present in the sera of thyrotoxic patients are directed against a site on the TSH receptor which produces the changes required for adenyl cyclase activation, just like TSH itself.

Learning Response D: Incorrect. Autoantibodies to the acetylcholine receptor are present in patients with myasthenia gravis. These antibodies induce the stripping of the receptors from the muscle end-plate and are an example of type II hypersensitivity.

Learning Response E: Incorrect. Thyroxine is one of the thyroid hormones. Although autoantibodies against this hormone have been described, they do not cause a type V hypersensitivity.

342. SUBJECT AREA: Core revision
QUESTION: Septic shock associated with Gram-negative bacteria is primarily due to:

- A: Lipopolysaccharide
- B: Enterotoxin superantigen
- C: Platelet aggregation
- D: Switch off of cytokine release
- E: Peptidoglycans

☐ Correct Answer: A

Learning Response A: Correct. Septicemia associated with Gram-negative bacteria results primarily from excessive release of tumor necrosis factor (TNF), IL-1 and IL-6, through stimulation of macrophages and endothelial cells by the lipopolysaccharide (LPS) endotoxin.

Learning Response B: Incorrect. Enterotoxin superantigens are associated with Gram-positive organisms and stimulate selected T cell families.

Learning Response C: Incorrect. *S. aureus* mediated aggregation of platelets induces disseminated intravascular coagulation.

Learning Response D: Incorrect. In septic shock associated with Gram-negative bacteria there is excessive release of TNF, IL-1 and IL-6 through stimulation of macrophages and endothelial cells.

Learning Response E: Incorrect. Peptidoglycans are Gram-positive cell wall components which are able to cause platelet aggregation.

343. SUBJECT AREA: Immunological basis of graft rejection
QUESTION: A graft between members of the same species is termed a(n):

- A: Autograft
- B: Isograft
- C: Xenograft
- D: Allograft
- E: None of the above

☐ Correct Answer: D

Learning Response A: Incorrect. An autograft is a graft from one part of the same individual to another.

Learning Response B: Incorrect. Isografts are grafts between identical members of the same species, e.g., identical twins or inbred strain mice.

Learning Response C: Incorrect. Xenografts refer to grafts between members of different species.

Learning Response D: Correct. These represent the most vigorous grafts because there are very high numbers of T cells with appropriate specificities.

Learning Response E: Incorrect.

---

344. SUBJECT AREA: Immunological basis of graft rejection
QUESTION: One of the following statements is false. Rejection of a second (set) skin graft from the same allogeneic donor:

    A: Can be blocked by azathioprine (an antimitotic agent)
    B: Proceeds at the same speed as the first graft rejection
    C: Shows specificity for the graft donor
    D: Can be transferred to a naive recipient with lymphocytes
    E: Cannot be transferred to a naive recipient with serum antibody

☐ Correct Answer: *B*

Learning Response A: Incorrect. This is a true statement. Azathioprine as an antimitotic agent blocks clonal proliferation and is often used as a therapeutic immunosuppressive agent.

Learning Response B: Correct. This is a false statement since the second graft is rejected far more rapidly due to immunological memory.

Learning Response C: Incorrect. This is a true statement.

Learning Response D: Incorrect. This is a true statement. T lymphocytes are involved.

Learning Response E: Incorrect. This is a true statement.

345. SUBJECT AREA: Transplantation antigens
QUESTION: The human major histocompatibility complex:

- *A:* Provokes the most intense allograft reactions
- *B:* Is termed H-2
- *C:* Contains only class I and class II genes
- *D:* Are not expressed as codominant antigens on the cell surface
- *E:* Are not associated with 'minor' transplantation antigens

☐ Correct Answer: *A*

Learning Response A: Correct. The MHC was recognized by its ability to produce the most intense graft rejection between members of the same species.

Learning Response B: Incorrect. H-2 is the MHC of the mouse.

Learning Response C: Incorrect. Range of class III genes are present within the MHC and include genes coding for components of the alternative pathway, C4, C2, TNF, TAP transporter genes for class I peptides and LMP2/7 associated with proteosome processing of cytosol proteins.

Learning Response D: Incorrect. Antigens from each parental haplotype are equally expressed on the cell surface.

Learning Response E: Incorrect. The minor transplantation antigens are processed peptides which associate with the MHC molecules on the cell surface and provide less potent graft antigens than the MHC themselves.

346. SUBJECT AREA: MHC incompatibility
QUESTION: Mitosis occurs when mixing lymphocytes of two individuals:

- *A:* In presence of mitomycin C
- *B:* In presence of anti-CD4
- *C:* Who are identical twins
- *D:* Of differing MHC class II haplotype
- *E:* Of differing MHC class I, but identical MHC class II, haplotype

☐ Correct Answer: *D*

Learning Response A: Incorrect. Mitomycin C inhibits cell division.

Learning Response B: Incorrect. Anti-CD4 blocks recognition by T-cell receptors.

Learning Response C: Incorrect. Identical twins have identical MHC class II haplotype.

Learning Response D: Correct. The mixed lymphocyte reaction is used for typing MHC class II polymorphic variants.

Learning Response E: Incorrect. Since the lymphocytes have identical MHC class II, there is no mixed lymphocyte reaction.

347. SUBJECT AREA: MHC incompatibility
QUESTION: Graft vs host disease occurs on injecting adult T cells of strain A into:

- *A:* F1 (A × B) animals
- *B:* Unirradiated strain B
- *C:* Irradiated strain A
- *D:* Strain A fetuses
- *E:* Cultures of lymphocytes from strain B

☐ Correct Answer: *A*

Learning Response A: Correct. F1 (A × B) animals will codominantly express the antigens of the A & B parents and the adult T cells of strain A, not being tolerant to the B antigens, will react against them and cause graft vs host disease.

Learning Response B: Incorrect. Strain B being unirradiated, will be capable of mounting a host vs graft reaction against the injected T cells of strain A.

Learning Response C: Incorrect. T cells on injection will be in the same genetic environment as the donor and would only see the host antigens as self.

Learning Response D: Incorrect. As in answer C, the adult T cells will be in a fully syngeneic environment and will not react against the host.

Learning Response E: Incorrect. There will be a mixed lymphocyte reaction but this is not the same as graft vs host disease which occurs in vivo.

348. SUBJECT AREA: Prevention of graft rejection
QUESTION: The MLR using homozygous stimulating cells, tissue types for antigens encoded by HLA-:

A: A
B: B
C: C
D: D
E: None of the above

☐ Correct Answer: *D*

Learning Response A: Incorrect. HLA-A encodes MHC class I antigens.

Learning Response B: Incorrect. HLA-B encodes MHC class I antigens.

Learning Response C: Incorrect. HLA-C encodes MHC class I antigens.

Learning Response D: Correct. The differences at the class II locus incite the mixed lymphocyte reaction. The cells to be typed come from an individual lacking the antigens present on the homozygous stimulating cells, there will be a mixed lymphocyte reaction.

Learning Response E: Incorrect.

349. SUBJECT AREA: Prevention of graft rejection
QUESTION: Non-specific suppression of graft rejection can be achieved with:

A: Ricin A chain
B: Anti-IL-5
C: Anti-NFκB
D: Anti-CD34
E: Anti-CD3

☐ Correct Answer: *E*

Learning Response A: Incorrect. Ricin A chain is only a toxin when it enters the cell usually attached to the ricin B chain which binds to receptors on the cell surface. Ricin A linked to certain antibodies which can be taken into cells by phagocytosis provides so-called magic bullets.

Learning Response B: Incorrect. Anti-IL-5 would block the eosinophilic responses to worm infestation and late phase allergic responses.

Learning Response C: Incorrect. Antibodies to the intracellular transcription factor NFκB cannot reach their antigen.

Learning Response D: Incorrect. CD34 is a marker of bone marrow stem cells.

Learning Response E: Correct. Anti-CD3 blocks TCR recognition of antigen and can also deplete T cells.

350. SUBJECT AREA: Prevention of graft rejection
QUESTION: The immunosuppressive drug which acts by alkylating and cross-linking DNA is:

- *A:* Azathioprine
- *B:* Cyclophosphamide
- *C:* Cyclosporin
- *D:* Rapamycin
- *E:* Prednisone

☐ Correct Answer: *B*

Learning Response A: Incorrect. Azathioprine is metabolized to a competitive antagonist of DNA synthesis.

Learning Response B: Correct.

Learning Response C: Incorrect. Cyclosporin blocks the formation of the transcription factors which control interleukin-2 expression.

Learning Response D: Incorrect. Rapamycin complexes with the FK-506 binding protein and blocks the activation of p70 S6 kinase by transduced IL-2 signals, thereby inhibiting cell division.

Learning Response E: Incorrect. Steroids affect lymphocyte recirculation, the generation of cytotoxic T cells, inhibit neutrophil adherence to endothelial cells and suppress the microbicidal activity of mononuclear phagocytes.

351. SUBJECT AREA: Prevention of graft rejection
QUESTION: An $H-2^k$ mouse is grafted with $H-2^b$ skin under anti-CD4/8 treatment. Which of the following grafts is rejected most rapidly:

A: H-2^k
B: The first H-2^b graft
C: A second H-2^b graft
D: An H-2^{bxk} graft
E: Third party H-2^a

☐ Correct Answer: *E*

Learning Response A: Incorrect. H-2^k would be a syngeneic graft whose antigens were identical with those of the host.

Learning Response B: Incorrect. The first H-2^b graft would induce tolerance through anti-CD4/8 treatment.

Learning Response C: Incorrect. Since the treatment with H-2^b graft under anti-CD4/8 treatment would induce tolerance, the second graft would not be rejected.

Learning Response D: Incorrect. The H-2^{bxk} graft would contain antigens encoded by both H-2^b and H-2^k. The host is tolerant to H-2^b because of the anti-CD4/8 treatment accompanying the H-2^b graft. H-2^k is a self-antigen so there would be no rejection of the graft.

Learning Response E: Correct. There would be no tolerance to H-2^a so this would be rejected as a first set graft and would be faster than all the other grafts which for various reasons would be accepted.

352. SUBJECT AREA: Clinical grafting
QUESTION: The 1-year survival rate for cadaver kidneys grafted into individuals pretreated with blood transfusion and with no DR mismatches is approximately:

A: 100%
B: 90%
C: 60%
D: 40%
E: 20%

☐ Correct Answer: *B*

Learning Response A: Incorrect.

Learning Response B: Correct. The beneficial effect of blood transfusion on graft survival is well recognized but the mechanism not understood. DR mismatches are the most disadvantageous for graft survival since differences at the HLA-D loci produce powerful T-cell activation seen in culture as the mixed lymphocyte reaction.

Learning Response C: Incorrect.

Learning Response D: Incorrect.

Learning Response E: Incorrect.

353. SUBJECT AREA: Clinical grafting
QUESTION: Graft vs host disease often accompanies transplantation of:

- *A:* Cartilage
- *B:* Kidney
- *C:* Bone marrow
- *D:* Heart
- *E:* Pancreas

☐ Correct Answer: *C*

Learning Response A: Incorrect. Cartilage has no adult T cells.

Learning Response B: Incorrect. Kidney has few if any adult T cells.

Learning Response C: Correct. Bone marrow usually has appreciable numbers of adult immunocompetent T cells capable of recognizing the transplantation antigens of the host and reacting against them causing graft versus host disease.

Learning Response D: Incorrect. Heart has no T cells.

Learning Response E: Incorrect. Pancreas has no T cells.

354. SUBJECT AREA: HLA & disease
QUESTION: The undue tendency for closely linked genes on a chromosome to remain associated rather than undergo genetic randomisation, is termed:

- *A:* Tandem duplication
- *B:* Meiotic crossover
- *C:* Relative risk

D: Linkage disequilibrium
E: Gene conversion

☐ Correct Answer: *D*

Learning Response A: Incorrect. Tandem duplication involves duplication of an existing gene and its insertion into the genome.

Learning Response B: Incorrect. Meiotic crossover involves interchange of genetic information between sister chromatids during myosis.

Learning Response C: Incorrect. Relative risk refers to the chance of developing a particular disease if one possesses a certain allele compared to the chance of developing disease if one has a different allele at the same locus.

Learning Response D: Correct. As a result of linkage disequilibrium, a disease associated with a particular gene could also show an association with a second gene which was in linkage disequilibrium with the first.

Learning Response E: Incorrect. Gene conversion involves the use of the DNA strand of the normal allele to repair a mutant gene sequence. Also used in species such as the chicken, to generate diversity in Ig genes.

355. Subject Area: HLA & disease
Question: DR2 is a risk factor for:

A: Multiple sclerosis
B: Insulin-dependent diabetes
C: Post-yersinia arthritis
D: Rheumatoid arthritis
E: Myasthenia gravis

☐ Correct Answer: *A*

Learning Response A: Correct. Individuals with DR2 are more at risk of developing multiple sclerosis than those with other DR specificities. Thus a higher frequency of DR2 is found in MS patients versus the normal population.

Learning Response B: Incorrect. DR3 and DR4 are risk factors for insulin-dependent diabetes.

Learning Response C: Incorrect. HLA-B27 is a powerful risk factor for post-yersinia arthritis.

Learning Response D: Incorrect. DR4 is a risk factor for rheumatoid arthritis.

Learning Response E: Incorrect. HLA-B8 is a risk factor for myasthenia gravis.

---

356. SUBJECT AREA: Reproductive immunology
QUESTION: HLA-G:

    A: Is an MHC class II molecule
    B: Is present on extravillous trophoblast
    C: Stimulates NK cell-mediated lysis
    D: Activates DAF
    E: Stimulates IL-10 synthesis

☐ Correct Answer: *B*

Learning Response A: Incorrect. HLA-G is a non-classical class I molecule.

Learning Response B: Correct. HLA-G present on the extravillous trophoblast membranes inhibits NK cell lysis and being non-polymorphic, is not a target for cytotoxic T cells.

Learning Response C: Incorrect. HLA-G inhibits NK cell activity.

Learning Response D: Incorrect. DAF is present independently on the trophoblast membranes and helps to break down any adventitiously formed C3 convertase which could lead to complement mediated damage.

Learning Response E: Incorrect. IL-10 is synthesized independent of HLA-G and acts to inhibit the generation of the inflammatory T_{h1} subset.

---

357. SUBJECT AREA: Fetal immunology
QUESTION: One of the following lacks the potential to be a candidate for an immunological contraceptive vaccine:

    A: LHRH
    B: Progesterone
    C: Estradiol
    D: hCG
    E: Human β-hCG + ovine α-chain

☐ Correct Answer: *C*

Learning Response A: Incorrect. LHRH is a potential candidate because antibodies to it will block release of luteinizing hormone which is essential for maturation of the female egg.

Learning Response B: Incorrect. Progesterone is a potential candidate since blocking by antibodies would prevent the maintenance of the fertile egg.

Learning Response C: Correct. Estradiol would not be a candidate since it is not involved in the maintenance of the fertile egg.

Learning Response D: Incorrect. hCG is an excellent candidate since antibodies would inhibit its action in maintaining the fertilized egg by stimulating progesterone release from the corpus luteum.

Learning Response E: Incorrect. As for answer D, hCG itself is an excellent candidate, the β-chain being specific for hCG. Combining with the ovine α-chain maintains the configuration of the β-subunit and also provides powerful helper epitopes.

---

358. SUBJECT AREA: Fetal immunology
QUESTION: An hCG vaccine is a good potential immunological contraceptive because hCG:

A: α-chain cross-reacts with other pituitary hormones
B: Is present in the male
C: Is vital for establishment of pregnancy
D: Is present throughout the menstrual cycle
E: Induces immunological tolerance

☐ Correct Answer: *C*

Learning Response A: Incorrect. The cross-reaction of the α-chain with other pituitary hormones, will produce unwanted neutralizing actions on hormones such as TSH.

Learning Response B: Incorrect. hCG is only present in the female at the time of pregnancy. Is not present in the male.

Learning Response C: Correct. hCG stimulates production of progesterone from the corpus luteum which is required for maintenance of the fertilized egg in the uterus.

Learning Response D: Incorrect. It is only present at the time of pregnancy and were it present throughout the menstrual cycle, it would be less desirable as a potential immunological contraceptive.

Learning Response E: Incorrect. hCG does not induce tolerance of B-cell epitopes because given an appropriate carrier, hCG can induce autoantibodies. If it did induce immunological tolerance, it would not be possible to induce the antibodies which would neutralize the hCG.

359. SUBJECT AREA: Core revision
QUESTION: The very rapid response to a *second* allogeneic graft is:

- A: Specific for antigens of the major histocompatibility complex (MHC)
- B: Dependent on minor histocompatibility antigens
- C: Transferred by macrophages to a naive recipient
- D: Transferred by platelets
- E: Transferred by IgA

☐ Correct Answer: A

Learning Response A: Correct. The very rapid second set response is obtained with antigens of the major histocompatibility complex and has memory for the antigens specific for the first graft.

Learning Response B: Incorrect. Antigens of the major histocompatibility complex are responsible for the fastest and most vigorous rejection of grafts between members of the same species. Other antigens termed minor histocompatibility antigens do give a faster second set graft rejection but this is not a *very rapid* response like that to the major histocompatibility antigens.

Learning Response C: Incorrect. Second set rejection can only be transferred by T-cells.

Learning Response D: Incorrect. Rejection of solid grafts is by T cells.

Learning Response E: Incorrect. IgA is not an inflammatory Ig.

360. SUBJECT AREA: Core revision
QUESTION: Concerning MHC class II antigen differences between 2 individuals, which of the following is *untrue*:

A: They produce mixed lymphocyte reactions
B: They stimulate formation of helpers to generate cytotoxic T cells
C: They cause graft vs host disease
D: For sibling pairs, they will only exist on average in 1:4 cases
E: None of the above

☐ Correct Answer: *D*

Learning Response A: Incorrect. This statement is true.

Learning Response B: Incorrect. This statement is true.

Learning Response C: Incorrect. This statement is true.

Learning Response D: Correct. This statement is untrue. Each parent contributes 2 different haplotypes giving a total possible combination of 4 different phenotypes. There is therefore a 1:4 chance that siblings would have identical phenotypes for class II.

Learning Response E: Incorrect.

361. SUBJECT AREA: Core revision
QUESTION: Hyperacute graft rejection is caused by:

A: Preformed antibody
B: CD4 lymphocytes
C: CD8 lymphocytes
D: Platelets
E: Circulating immune complexes

☐ Correct Answer: *A*

Learning Response A: Correct. Rejection occurs within minutes and is usually due to blood group incompatibility not presensitization to class I MHC through blood transfusion.

Learning Response B: Incorrect. CD4 lymphocytes contribute to rejection of solid grafts.

Learning Response C: Incorrect. CD8 lymphocytes may contribute to rejection of solid grafts.

Learning Response D: Incorrect. Platelet thrombin may be involved in acute late rejection of human renal allografts following deposition of antibody on the glomerular vessel wall.

Learning Response E: Incorrect. Complexes may be involved in the insidious and late rejection associated with subendothelial deposits of Ig and C3 on glomerular basement membranes.

---

362. SUBJECT AREA: Core revision
QUESTION: Which of the following *does not* minimize allogeneic graft rejection:

- A: Cyclosporin
- B: AZT
- C: Azathioprine
- D: Cross-matching for ABO and MHC
- E: Anti-CD4

☐ Correct Answer: *B*

Learning Response A: Incorrect. Cyclosporin with cyclophilin blocks the phosphatase which activates the NFAT transcription factor for the IL-2 enhancer.

Learning Response B: Correct. AZT inhibits the HIV reverse transcriptase and has nothing to do with graft rejection.

Learning Response C: Incorrect. Azathioprine is an antimitotic agent that blocks DNA synthesis by forming a metabolic antagonist.

Learning Response D: Incorrect. Matching for ABO and MHC improves graft survival.

Learning Response E: Incorrect. Anti-CD4 inhibits the activation of T cells by the graft.

---

363. SUBJECT AREA: Core revision
QUESTION: Which of the following allogeneic grafts *does not* require immunosuppression:

- A: Kidney
- B: Heart
- C: Liver

D: Bone marrow
E: Cartilage

☐ Correct Answer: *E*

Learning Response A: Incorrect.

Learning Response B: Incorrect.

Learning Response C: Incorrect.

Learning Response D: Incorrect.

Learning Response E: Correct. They are avascular and do not sensitize the recipient; the matrix also protects the chondrocytes.

364. SUBJECT AREA: Core Revision
QUESTION: Ankylosing spondylitis is strongly associated with HLA-:

A: B8
B: DR3
C: DR4
D: B27
E: DR2

☐ Correct Answer: *D*

Learning Response A: Incorrect. B8 is a risk factor for myasthenia gravis.

Learning Response B: Incorrect. DR3 is a risk factor for Addison's disease, insulin-dependent diabetes, etc.

Learning Response C: Incorrect. DR4 is a risk factor for rheumatoid arthritis and insulin-dependent diabetes.

Learning Response D: Correct. The relative risk of developing this disease in B27 positive individuals is 87.4.

Learning Response E: Incorrect. DR2 is a risk factor for multiple sclerosis and Goodpasture's syndrome but a protective factor for insulin-dependent diabetes.

365. SUBJECT AREA: Core revision
QUESTION: The fetus is protected from maternal transplantation attack by:

    A: Luteinizing hormone
    B: Lack of HLA class I on the fetus
    C: HLA-G on the extravillous cytotrophoblast
    D: C3 convertase on the syncitiotrophoblast
    E: Local production of IL-2

☐ Correct Answer: *C*

Learning Response A: Incorrect. Luteinizing hormone aids the maturation of the female oocyte.

Learning Response B: Incorrect. There is a lack of classical HLA class I on the fetal membranes but this is replaced by the non-classical HLA-G which is not susceptible to attack by cytotoxic lymphocytes and also inhibits the activity of NK cells.

Learning Response C: Correct. The non-classical HLA-G which is not susceptible to attack by cytotoxic lymphocytes and also inhibits the activity of NK cells.

Learning Response D: Incorrect. There are, however, molecules such as DAF which inhibit the activity of any complement components deposited on the fetal membranes.

Learning Response E: Incorrect. There is production of cytokines such as TGF-β which is immunosuppressive and IL-10 which inhibits the activity of the inflammatory T_{h1} subset.

366. SUBJECT AREA: Core revision
QUESTION: The normal immunological control of tumors is referred to as:

    A: Immunological tolerance
    B: Immune surveillance
    C: Type III hypersensitivity
    D: Immunological silence
    E: Superantigen recognition

☐ Correct Answer: *B*

Learning Response A: Incorrect. This is a mechanism which prevents immune reactivity, for example against self antigens, and thus would not be helpful in the immunological control of tumors.

Learning Response B: Correct. Immunological surveillance refers to the recognition of altered cells with a neoplastic potential which may then be eliminated to prevent the emergence of the tumor.

Learning Response C: Incorrect. These are immune-complex mediated hypersensitivity reactions as seen in, for example, glomerulonephritis in the autoimmune disease systemic lupus erythematosus (SLE).

Learning Response D: Incorrect. This refers to immunological nonreactivity, for example against largely sequestered (hidden) self antigens such as is thought to be the case for lens, sperm and brain antigens.

Learning Response E: Incorrect. Superantigens are those that bind to particular T cell receptor Vβ sequences irrespective of the D and J regions, or the α chain, that is used. They thus stimulate a much greater proportion of T cells than would be the case with conventional antigen. Examples include *Staphylococcus* enterotoxin B (SEB) and murine Mls.

---

367. SUBJECT AREA: Changes on the surface of tumor cells
QUESTION: An example of a known oncogenic virus is:

- *A:* Herpes zoster
- *B:* HIV-2
- *C:* Epstein-Barr virus
- *D:* Vesicular stomatitis virus
- *E:* Proteus mirabilis

☐ Correct Answer: *C*

Learning Response A: Incorrect. These particular herpesviruses are not oncogenic. Herpes zoster causes chickenpox, and when reactivated in adulthood causes shingles.

Learning Response B: Incorrect. This virus, as well as the more prevalent HIV-1, is the causative agent of acquired immune deficiency syndrome (AIDS).

Learning Response C: Correct. Epstein-Barr virus is associated with Burkitt's lymphoma and with naso-pharyngeal carcinoma.

Learning Response D: Incorrect. Vesicular stomatosis is a non-malignant infectious disease of domestic animals in the Americas.

Learning Response E: Incorrect. *Proteus mirabilis* is not a virus, but a Gram negative bacterium which has been postulated as an etiological agent in the autoimmune disease rheumatoid arthritis through molecular mimicry with HLA-DR4/DR1 self antigen.

---

368. SUBJECT AREA: Core revision
QUESTION: Antigens normally expressed only on embryonic cells but also sometimes found on tumors are known as:

   A: Oncofetal antigens
   B: HTLV-1
   C: Maternal
   D: Neonatal
   E: Cryptic

☐ Correct Answer: *A*

Learning Response A: Correct. Dysregulated uncontrolled cell division of the cancer cell may be associated with the expression of products of normally silent genes such as those encoding differentiation antigens normally associated with the earlier fetal stage.

Learning Response B: Incorrect. Human T-cell lymphotropic virus type 1 (HTLV-1) is associated with a subset of adult human T-cell leukemia. After infection of the T cell, the viral tax protein stimulates transcription of interleukin-2 (IL-2), IL-2 receptor and other growth factors leading to vigorous proliferation. Only if there is a subsequent chromosomal translocation does malignant transformation take place.

Learning Response C: Incorrect. The term maternal refers to antigen expressed by, or derived from, the mother.

Learning Response D: Incorrect. The neonatal period refers to the first few weeks post-partum. A time of rapid development of the baby's immune system which needs to provide protection against a harsh microbiological environment, a battle fought alone once the maternally-derived IgG is catabolised and thus disappears from the baby's circulation. In breast fed offspring, further help can be found in the form of maternal secretory IgA.

Learning Response E: Incorrect. Cryptic epitopes are those which do not normally reach a critical concentration on professional antigen-presenting cells to stimulate resting naive T cells, for example, those which are largely sequestered from the immune system, not produced in abundance by intracellular processor or with poor affinity for the MHC groove.

369. SUBJECT AREA: Changes on the surface of tumor cells
QUESTION: In pancreatic carcinoma the *ras* gene:

- *A:* Is absent
- *B:* Is normal but is overexpressed
- *C:* Has a large deletion
- *D:* Contains a single point mutation, always at the same position
- *E:* Contains a single point mutation, but not always at the same position

☐ Correct Answer: *E*

Learning Response A: Incorrect. *Ras* is present in both normal subjects and in patients with pancreatic carcinoma. However, in the latter group the gene is altered.

Learning Response B: Incorrect. The oncogenic human *ras* genes differ structurally from their normal counterpart.

Learning Response C: Incorrect. The oncogenic human *ras* genes do not contain either large deletions or insertions.

Learning Response D: Incorrect. Almost right!

Learning Response E: Correct. A point mutation leads to a single amino acid substitution at either position 12, 13 or 61. These mutations are found in over 90% of patients with pancreatic carcinomas, in 40% of patients with colorectal cancers and their preneoplastic lesions, in acute myeloid leukemia (AML) and in preleukemic syndromes.

370. SUBJECT AREA: Changes on the surface of tumor cells
QUESTION: Wheat germ agglutinin binds strongly to:

- *A:* Surface lipoproteins on resting T cells
- *B:* Surface glycoproteins on resting T cells

C: Surface glycoproteins on resting B cells
D: Surface glycoproteins on activated T and B cells
E: Surface lipoproteins on activated T and B cells

☐ Correct Answer: *D*

Learning Response A: Incorrect. Wheat germ agglutinin is a plant lectin which recognizes specific sugars on oligosaccharides and therefore would not bind to lipoproteins.

Learning Response B: Incorrect. Wheat germ agglutinin does bind to glycoproteins but the sugars it recognizes are poorly represented on the cell surface of resting T cells.

Learning Response C: Incorrect. Wheat germ agglutinin does bind to glycoproteins but the sugars it recognizes are poorly represented on the cell surface of resting B cells.

Learning Response D: Correct. Within 24 hours of stimulation by lymphocyte polyclonal activators, high concentrations of binding sites for this lectin appear on the surface of the cell.

Learning Response E: Incorrect. Wheat germ agglutinin is a plant lectin which recognizes specific sugars on oligosaccharides and therefore would not bind to lipoproteins.

---

371. SUBJECT AREA: Immune response to tumors
QUESTION: Boon and colleagues showed that syngeneic transplantable tumors which mutate such that they express strong transplantation antigens are rejected. They called these variants:

A: tum^-
B: Xenogeneic
C: tum^+
D: MCA
E: Non-immunogenic

☐ Correct Answer: *A*

Learning Response A: Correct. Tum^- cell lines are those which have mutated such that they cannot be grown in syngeneic animals with a normal immune system.

Learning Response B: Incorrect. The term xenogeneic refers to the genetic differences between species, and therefore by definition xenogeneic tumors are not syngeneic.

Learning Response C: Incorrect. Tum^+ refers to the parental tumor cells which can be passaged within a pure mouse strain without provoking rejection.

Learning Response D: Incorrect. Methylcholanthrene (MCA) is a chemical carcinogen which Prehn and Main used to demonstrate clearly that chemically-induced cancers can trigger immune responses to themselves but not to other tumors produced by the same carcinogen.

Learning Response E: Incorrect. The fact that they are actively rejected means that they are immunogenic.

---

372. SUBJECT AREA: Core revision
QUESTION: CD44 is a molecule which may be involved in:

- *A:* Neoplastic transformation
- *B:* Metastatic spread
- *C:* Tumor surveillance
- *D:* Antigen recognition
- *E:* Secretion of tumor necrosis factor

☐ Correct Answer: *B*

Learning Response A: Incorrect. CD44 (HERMES/Pgp-1) is a normally expressed adhesion molecule involved in cell trafficking based on its interaction with vascular endothelium.

Learning Response B: Correct. CD44 (HERMES/Pgp-1) is an adhesion molecule involved in cell trafficking based on its interaction with vascular endothelium. It occurs in several isoforms and normal colon epithelium is largely negative for the V6 exon-encoded sequence which is expressed much more frequently in tumors.

Learning Response C: Incorrect. CD44 is a normal cell surface antigen involved in adhesion to vascular endothelium and therefore would not be distinguished by immune surveillance mechanisms seeking out rogue tumor-associated antigens.

Learning Response D: Incorrect. The only molecules concerned in antigen recognition are immunoglobulin, the T-cell receptor, and MHC. Immunoglobulin and the T-cell receptor are highly specific, MHC has a much broader specificity recognizing a larger number of different peptides which possess the relevant anchor amino acids to fit into pockets in the MHC groove.

Learning Response E: Incorrect. There is no evidence for any direct role of CD44 in TNF secretion. Note that the main function of TNF is as an inflammatory cytokine, although as its name suggests it can cause the necrosis of some tumors.

373. SUBJECT AREA: Core revision

QUESTION: A B-cell lymphoma will express a unique tumor antigen called:

A: p53
B: Endosialin
C: SM-3
D: Idiotype
E: Lewis Le^a

☐ Correct Answer: *D*

Learning Response A: Incorrect. p53 is a cell cycle inhibitor which in many tumors shows single point mutations.

Learning Response B: Incorrect. Endosialin is a highly sialylated cell surface glycoprotein (FB5) present in the vasculature of a significant proportion of malignant tumors but not in the blood vessels of normal tissues.

Learning Response C: Incorrect. SM-3 is a monoclonal antibody, directed to the core polypeptide of pancreatic and breast mucins, which reacts poorly with normal tissue where the epitope is masked by abundant O-linked carbohydrate chains, but reacts well with the less glycosylated versions of these mucins which are associated with tumors.

Learning Response D: Correct. This opens up the possibility of making a highly-specific tumor vaccine or anti-tumor therapeutic agent. In fact B-cell lymphomas have been successfully treated using anti-idiotypes. One (of several) major difficulties is that the reagents need to be tailored to each individual's idiotype.

Learning Response E: Incorrect. Lewis Le^a is a normal antigen abnormally expressed on some gastrointestinal cancers in individuals who are Le(a$^-$,b$^-$).

374. SUBJECT AREA: Immune response to tumors

QUESTION: Strongly immunogenic tumors appear:

A: In virtually all cancers

B: Only in lymphoma and leukemia
C: In immunosuppressed patients
D: Only in experimental animals
E: Only in elderly patients

☐ Correct Answer: *C*

Learning Response A: Incorrect. If all tumors were strongly immunogenic, one might hope that the incidence of cancer would be much lower than it is.

Learning Response B: Incorrect. Epstein-Barr virus (EBV)-positive lymphomas are potentially strongly immunogenic, but most normal individuals have highly efficient EBV-specific cytotoxic T lymphocytes (CTL) suggesting perhaps that the lymphoma cells downregulate cell surface molecules that might be targets for the CTL.

Learning Response C: Correct. For example, skin cancers and lymphomas seen in transplant patients receiving immunosuppression.

Learning Response D: Incorrect. Although chemically-induced tumors in mice are often highly immunogenic it is thought that many human tumors are also 'nipped in the bud' due to their innate immunogenicity, e.g., skin cancers.

Learning Response E: Incorrect. In children with Wiskott-Aldrich syndrome there is a T-cell deficiency and this is associated with an increased incidence of potentially strongly immunogenic lymphomas. These patients show an unusually restricted expression of EBV latent proteins which are the major potential target epitopes for immune recognition.

375. SUBJECT AREA: Immune response to tumors
QUESTION: A mouse strain deficient in NK cells is the:

A: SJL
B: Beige
C: Nude
D: MRL-*lpr/lpr*
E: Moth-eaten viable

☐ Correct Answer: *B*

Learning Response A: Incorrect. SJL mice do, however, appear to have defective T-cell mediated suppressor mechanisms and are thus potentially susceptible to certain forms of induced autoimmune disease such as autoimmune hemolytic anemia (AHA) triggered by injection of cross-reactive rat erythrocytes.

Learning Response B: Correct. NK cells are spontaneously cytolytic for certain tumor cell lines and express CD16, the low affinity FcγRIII. Beige mice congenitally lack type I NK cells and die with spontaneous tumors earlier than their non-deficient heterozygous +/*bg* littermates.

Learning Response C: Incorrect. Nude mice are congenitally athymic and therefore lack mature T cells. They are also hairless, hence their name.

Learning Response D: Incorrect. MRL strain mice homozygous for the lymphoproliferation (*lpr*) gene (a mutation in the *Fas* gene) have a massive polyclonal proliferation of an unusual T-cell population, leading to massive lymphadenopathy and autoimmune phenomena reminiscent of those seen in some human rheumatological disorders such as rheumatoid arthritis and SLE.

Learning Response E: Incorrect. The moth-eaten viable (Me^V) mouse is an animal model of immunodeficiency involving impaired T, B and NK cell function associated with a *hyper*gammaglobulinemia.

---

376. SUBJECT AREA: Unregulated development gives rise to lymphoproliferative disorders
QUESTION: Which of the following is most commonly seen in African children with Burkitt's lymphoma:

A: Absence of EBV
B: T-cell neoplasia
C: Deletion of the *c-myc* gene
D: Chromosome 8q24 to Chromosome 14q32 translocation
E: Chromosome 8q24 to Chromosome 2p12 translocation

☐ Correct Answer: *D*

Learning Response A: Incorrect. Burkitt's lymphoma in Africa is strongly associated with EBV infection. This virus is also found in association with nasopharyngeal carcinoma in Japan and, worldwide, with infectious mononucleosis (glandular fever), a nonmalignant disease.

Learning Response B: Incorrect. Burkitt's lymphoma is a B-cell neoplasia.

Learning Response C: Incorrect. The *c-myc* gene is not deleted in Burkitt's lymphoma.

Learning Response D: Correct. The *c-myc* gene (chromosome 8q24) involved in the entry of cells from resting G_0 into the cell cycle is translocated to the μ heavy chain gene (chromosome 14q32) in most cases of Burkitt's lymphoma studied.

Learning Response E: Incorrect. The translocation of the *c-myc* gene (chromosome 8q24) to the immunoglobulin κ light chain gene (chromosome 2p12) is seen in some cases of Burkitt's lymphoma, but not the majority.

377. SUBJECT AREA: Core revision
QUESTION: Malignant lymphoid cells:

   A: Show maturation arrest at characteristic stages in differentiation
   B: Form a polyclonal population of cells
   C: Are non-dividing
   D: Express several different tumor-specific antigens
   E: Are always derived from various stages of the normal B-cell differentiation pathway

☐ Correct Answer: *A*

Learning Response A: Correct. Lymphoid cells at almost any stage in their differentiation or maturation may become malignant and proliferate to form a clone of cells which are 'frozen' at a particular stage of development.

Learning Response B: Incorrect. They are monoclonal, as shown by the fact that, in the case of B cells, they express either κ or λ light chains but not both, and they express a single idiotype.

Learning Response C: Incorrect. It is the characteristic of proliferation in an uncontrolled manner which makes these cells malignant.

Learning Response D: Incorrect. However, they do express idiotype which is effectively a tumor-specific marker as only the malignant clone will bear this particular idiotype, related to the original antigen-specificity of the parental T or B cell.

Learning Response E: Incorrect. Tumors of lymphoid cells are not limited to B lymphocytes but can also be derived from other lymphoid cells types, e.g., T-cell acute lymphoblastic leukemia (T-ALL).

378. SUBJECT AREA: Unregulated development gives rise to lymphoproliferative disorders

QUESTION: Chronic lymphocytic leukemia:

- *A:* Usually has a very poor prognosis
- *B:* Has a good prognosis only in those patients with circulating monoclonal immunoglobulin
- *C:* Is mostly a disease of childhood
- *D:* Is usually found in people over 50 years of age
- *E:* Is a leukemia where both κ and λ light chains are found on the surface of the malignant cell

☐ Correct Answer: *D*

Learning Response A: Incorrect. Chronic lymphocytic leukemia (CLL) is usually (but not always) relatively benign to the extent that in some patients it can be left untreated.

Learning Response B: Incorrect. The 10–20% of patients with chronic lymphocytic leukemia in whom there is circulating monoclonal immunoglobulin have a poor prognosis.

Learning Response C: Incorrect. Common acute lymphoblastic leukemia antigen (CALLA)-positive ALL is the most common leukemia in children, whereas CLL is uncommon in people under 50 years of age.

Learning Response D: Correct. CLL is uncommon in people under 50 years of age.

Learning Response E: Incorrect. Leukemias are monoclonal, i.e. derived from a neoplastic event in a single cell, therefore in a B-cell leukemia the light chain on the malignant cells will be either κ or λ but not both.

379. SUBJECT AREA: Unregulated development gives rise to lymphoproliferative disorders

QUESTION: Non-Hodgkin lymphomas:

- *A:* Will be positive when stained with antibodies to cytokeratin
- *B:* Are usually of T-cell origin but sometimes of B-cell origin
- *C:* Can be differentiated from carcinoma using antibodies to leukocyte common antigen
- *D:* Are reactive B-cell hyperplasias
- *E:* Have a good prognosis

☐ Correct Answer: *C*

Learning Response A: Incorrect. Antibodies to cytokeratin will recognize most carcinomas, not lymphomas.

Learning Response B: Incorrect. The majority of non-Hodgkin lymphomas are of B-cell origin.

Learning Response C: Correct. The sometimes difficult distinction between a lymphoproliferative condition and carcinoma can be made with ease by using monoclonal antibodies to the leukocyte common antigen (CD45) which will react with all lymphoid cells whether in paraffin or cryostat sections.

Learning Response D: Incorrect. Reactive B-cell hyperplasias are polyclonal, not monoclonal, as shown by expression of both κ and λ light chains on the proliferating cell populations. Non-Hodgkin lymphoma, being a lymphoid cell malignancy, is monoclonal.

Learning Response E: Incorrect. Overall non-Hodgkin lymphomas have a poor prognosis even though the prognosis has improved with the use of combined immunotherapy. These lymphomas are 35 times more likely to develop in transplant patients, but this may not be wholly attributable to long-term immunosuppression as previously was thought to be the case.

380. Subject Area: Core revision

QUESTION: The amyloid deposits found in 10–20% of patients with myeloma contain:

A: Immunoglobulin light chains
B: Immunoglobulin heavy chains
C: Amyloid A (AA) protein
D: Isolated single molecules
E: Congo red

☐ Correct Answer: *A*

Learning Response A: Correct. Immunoglobulin-secreting cells produce an excess of light chain over heavy chain. Fragments of this excess light chain forms the amyloid deposits found in 10–20% of patients with myeloma.

Learning Response B: Incorrect. Almost right, but not quite!

Learning Response C: Incorrect. Amyloid which is found secondarily to chronic inflammatory conditions such as rheumatoid arthritis and familial Mediterranean fever contains amyloid A (AA) protein derived from the N-terminal part of a 90kDa serum precursor called SAA.

Learning Response D: Incorrect. The amyloid deposits found in myeloma patients are polymers, not monomers.

Learning Response E: Incorrect. Congo red is a dye which can be used in the laboratory to detect amyloid fibrils.

---

381. SUBJECT AREA: Core revision
QUESTION: In Waldenström's macroglobulinemia there is secretion of:

> *A:* Polyclonal IgG
> *B:* Monoclonal IgG
> *C:* Polyclonal IgM
> *D:* Monoclonal IgM
> *E:* Monoclonal antibody of mixed class

☐ Correct Answer: *D*

Learning Response A: Incorrect. In Waldenström's macroglobulinemia there is secretion of a monoclonal antibody.

Learning Response B: Incorrect. In Waldenström's macroglobulinemia there is secretion of a monoclonal antibody, but not of the IgG isotype.

Learning Response C: Incorrect. In Waldenström's macroglobulinemia there is secretion of a monoclonal antibody.

Learning Response D: Correct. In Waldenström's macroglobulinemia there is a dysregulated proliferation of cells of an intermediate differentiation stage. Many of the monoclonal IgM antibodies secreted by these lymphoplasmacytoid cells in different patients have autoantibody activity, for example anti-DNA, rheumatoid factor (anti-IgG), etc.

Learning Response E: Incorrect. Monoclonal antibodies are virtually always of a single class.

382. SUBJECT AREA: Cancer therapy

QUESTION: In Burkitt's lymphoma, a vaccine against which of the following might prove useful:

   A: Epstein-Barr virus
   B: Marek's disease virus
   C: Papilloma virus
   D: HTLV-1
   E: MMTV

☐ Correct Answer: A

Learning Response A: Correct. In human Burkitt's lymphoma work is in progress to develop a vaccine to exploit the ability of cytotoxic T cells to target EBV-related antigens on the cells of all Burkitt's tumors. It may be an advantage to treat the patients at the same time with cytokines to upregulate the expression of ICAM-1, LFA-3 and possibly of the virus itself.

Learning Response B: Incorrect. Marek's disease is a lymphoma in chickens. Large scale protection of chickens has been successfully achieved by vaccination with another herpes virus native to chickens rather than with the Marek's disease virus itself.

Learning Response C: Incorrect. Infection with papilloma virus is thought to be associated with certain skin cancers in man.

Learning Response D: Incorrect. Human T-cell leukemia virus (HTLV-1) is closely linked to the production of a T-cell leukemia of high prevelance in Japan.

Learning Response E: Incorrect. MMTV is mouse mammary tumor virus which is transmitted as an infectious agent in milk and acts as a superantigen.

383. SUBJECT AREA: Cancer therapy

QUESTION: Bone marrow purging in myeloid leukemias can be successfully carried out using antibodies to:

   A: CD3
   B: CD33
   C: CD5
   D: CD45
   E: CD1

☐ Correct Answer: *B*

Learning Response A: Incorrect. CD3 is a marker of T cells, found in association with the T-cell receptor.

Learning Response B: Correct. Anti-CD33 is highly specific for myeloid leukemias in relation to other hematopoietic stem cells and has been used successfully for bone marrow purging and also for therapy.

Learning Response C: Incorrect. CD5 is a lymphoid cell marker found on virtually all T cells and on a subset of B cells.

Learning Response D: Incorrect. CD45 is the leukocyte common antigen which is broadly distributed on leukocytes.

Learning Response E: Incorrect. CD1 is a marker of thymocytes, Langerhans' cells and dendritic cells.

---

384. SUBJECT AREA: Core revision
QUESTION: The term LAK cells refers to activated:

- *A:* Polymorphonuclear leukocytes
- *B:* B cells
- *C:* Macrophages
- *D:* Mast cells
- *E:* NK cells

☐ Correct Answer: *E*

Learning Response A: Incorrect. LAK cells are lymphokine-activated killer cells, but these are not derived from PMNs.

Learning Response B: Incorrect. LAK stands for lymphokine-activated killer cells, but they are not activated B-cells.

Learning Response C: Incorrect. LAK stands for lymphokine-activated killer cells, but they are not activated macrophages.

Learning Response D: Incorrect. LAK cells are lymphokine-activated killer cells, but these are not derived from mast cells.

Learning Response E: Correct. NK cells activated in vitro with IL-2 are called lymphokine-activated killer (LAK) cells. In one study, LAK cells given therapeutically together with high dose IL-2 led to a considerable reduction in renal tumor mass.

385. SUBJECT AREA: Immunodiagnosis of solid tumors
QUESTION: A diagnostic marker for tumors of the colon is:

- A: α-fetoprotein
- B: Carcinoembryonic antigen (CEA)
- C: The presence of Reed-Sternberg cells
- D: EBV-related antigens
- E: CALLA

☐ Correct Answer: *B*

Learning Response A: Incorrect. α-fetoprotein is an oncofetal antigen which is a diagnostic marker for hepatoma.

Learning Response B: Correct. Carcinoembryonic antigen (CEA) is an oncofetal antigen but there is a high incidence of false positives. Reappearance of CEA after surgical removal of the primary tumor is strongly indicative of fresh tumor growth.

Learning Response C: Incorrect. The lineage of the Reed-Sternberg cells found in lymphoma is unclear, but they are probably of either T-cell or macrophage lineage. Feedback suppression influences on the normal counterpart would be consistent with defects in cell-mediated immunity in these patients.

Learning Response D: Incorrect. Epstein-Barr virus related antigens are present in patients with Burkitt's lymphoma.

Learning Response E: Incorrect. The common acute lymphoblastic leukemia antigen (CALLA) is expressed in childhood ALL.

386. SUBJECT AREA: Scope of autoimmune diseases
QUESTION: Which of the following is a non-organ-specific (systemic) autoimmune disease:

- A: Myasthenia gravis
- B: Systemic lupus erythematosus (SLE)
- C: Hashimoto's thyroiditis

D: Pernicious anemia
E: Juvenile (insulin-dependent) diabetes

☐ Correct Answer: *B*

Learning Response A: Incorrect. Myasthenia gravis involves the production of antibodies to the organ-specific antigen, the acetylcholine receptor present on the muscle endplate.

Learning Response B: Correct. SLE is a disease involving antibodies to non-organ specific antigens such as DNA and induces immune complexes which deposit in the vascular bed causing kidney, skin, joint and cerebral lesions.

Learning Response C: Incorrect. Hashimoto's thyroiditis involves organ-specific attack of inflammatory cells on the thyroid and production of anti-thyroglobulin and anti-thyroid peroxidase specific to the thyroid gland.

Learning Response D: Incorrect. Pernicious anemia involves organ-specific attack on the gastric mucosa with autoantibodies to the parietal cells and intrinsic factor.

Learning Response E: Incorrect. Insulin-dependent diabetes involves specific inflammatory cell attack on the β cells of the islets of Langerhans and the production of a range of autoantibodies reacting with pancreatic antigens.

387. SUBJECT AREA: Scope of autoimmune diseases
QUESTION: Which of the following antibodies are of most use for the diagnosis of pernicious anemia:

A: Anti-parietal cell
B: Anti-thyroid peroxidase
C: Anti-nuclear
D: Anti-IgG Fc
E: Anti-TSH receptor

☐ Correct Answer: *A*

Learning Response A: Correct. Parietal cell antibodies detected by immuno-fluorescence on stomach sections are important markers of inflammatory atrophic gastritis and the subsequent pernicious anemia which can develop. Antibodies to intrinsic factor are even stronger confirmation.

Learning Response B: Incorrect. Anti-thyroid peroxidase are markers of autoimmune thyroid disease, Hashimoto's thyroiditis and primary myxedema.

Learning Response C: Incorrect. Anti-nuclear antibodies are particularly prominent in the rheumatological disorders, and are particularly seen in SLE.

Learning Response D: Incorrect. Anti-IgG Fc are the rheumatoid factors which are an important feature of rheumatoid arthritis.

Learning Response E: Incorrect. Anti-TSH receptors are responsible for the stimulation of the thyroid in Graves' thyrotoxicosis but may also play a blocking role in primary myxedema.

388. SUBJECT AREA: Scope of autoimmune diseases
QUESTION: Which of the following antibodies are of most use for the diagnosis of Sjögren's syndrome:

A: Anti-cardiolipin
B: Anti-neutrophil cytoplasm (ANCA)
C: Anti-SS-A(Ro), anti-SS-B(La)
D: Anti-mitochondrial
E: Anti-glomerular basement membrane

☐ Correct Answer: *C*

Learning Response A: Incorrect. Anti-cardiolipin is seen in SLE and particularly in thrombotic episodes of the anti-phospholipid syndrome.

Learning Response B: Incorrect. ANCA are particularly characteristic of Wegener's granulomatosis.

Learning Response C: Correct. They give a speckled nuclear fluorescence pattern.

Learning Response D: Incorrect. Anti-mitochondrial antibodies feature prominently in primary biliary cirrhosis.

Learning Response E: Incorrect. Anti-GBM are characteristic of Goodpasture's syndrome.

389. SUBJECT AREA: Scope of autoimmune diseases
QUESTION: The disease most frequently seen in association with pernicious anemia is:

  A: Addison's disease of the adrenal
  B: Multiple sclerosis
  C: Autoimmune hemolytic anemia
  D: Rheumatoid arthritis
  E: Graves' thyrotoxicosis

☐ Correct Answer: *E*

Learning Response A: Incorrect. Although an autoimmune disease which can occur in association with other autoimmune diseases as in the multiendocrinopathies, Addison's disease of the adrenal is relatively rare.

Learning Response B: Incorrect. Multiple sclerosis is targetted to a specific organ, the brain, but does not appear in association with other organ-specific diseases. Could this be because there might be viral involvement in the etiopathogenesis?

Learning Response C: Incorrect. Autoimmune hemolytic anemia is allied more closely to the systemic autoimmunity and is not associated with organ-specific diseases.

Learning Response D: Incorrect. Rheumatoid arthritis is a member of the systemic autoimmune diseases which are non-organ specific.

Learning Response E: Correct. Graves' thyrotoxicosis is a fairly frequent organ-specific disease and is often found in association with PA.

390. SUBJECT AREA: Scope of autoimmune diseases
QUESTION: Which of the following models is an example of a spontaneous organ-specific autoimmune disease:

  A: (NZB x W)F1
  B: MRL/lpr
  C: Experimental autoallergic encephalomyelitis
  D: Thyroiditis induced by early thymectomy and irradiation
  E: Non-obese diabetic (NOD) mouse

☐ Correct Answer: *E*

Learning Response A: Incorrect. This is a spontaneous non-organ specific disease producing anti-DNA and immune complex glomerulonephritis.

Learning Response B: Incorrect. This is an example of a non-organ specific spontaneous disease producing anti-DNA and immune complex glomerulonephritis associated with intense proliferation of lymphocytes.

Learning Response C: Incorrect. This is an experimentally induced organ-specific disease produced by brain myelin basic protein in Complete Freund's adjuvant leading to autoallergic attack on the brain and demyelination.

Learning Response D: Incorrect. This is an induced not a spontaneous organ-specific autoimmune disease presumably resulting from a selective loss of suppressors of lymphocytes with self-reactivity for the thyroid.

Learning Response E: Correct. These mice spontaneously develop inflammatory attack on islets of Langerhans and the production of antibodies to a variety of islet cell antigens.

391. SUBJECT AREA: Nature and nurture
QUESTION: The high concordance rate for monozygotic vs dizygotic twins in type 1 diabetes indicates:

- *A:* A strong environmental element
- *B:* A strong genetic element
- *C:* A major influence of sex
- *D:* The influence of HLA
- *E:* The possibility of microbial infection

☐ Correct Answer: *B*

Learning Response A: Incorrect. If the concordance rate for non-identical dizygotic twins were the same as for genetically identical monozygotic twins, this would have been evidence for a strong environmental as distinct from a genetic element.

Learning Response B: Correct. The higher concordance rate for genetically identical monozygotic compared to the genetically non-identical dizygotic twins brought up in the same environment clearly favours a strong genetic element.

Learning Response C: Incorrect. The statement says nothing about sex since the twins can be randomly of either sex, except for identity between monozygotic twins.

Learning Response D: Incorrect. The statement indicates a strong genetic element but does not provide evidence for that being HLA which has to be established independently.

Learning Response E: Incorrect. The statement is against a major environmental influence and therefore against a possible microbial infection as a major factor.

---

392. SUBJECT AREA: Natural autoimmunity
QUESTION: Which of the following is *incorrect*. 'Natural antibodies' are often:

    A: Autoreactive
    B: Polyspecific
    C: Reactive with bacterial carbohydrates
    D: High affinity IgG
    E: Produced by $CD5^+$ B cells

☐ Correct Answer: *D*

Learning Response A: Incorrect. The statement is true.

Learning Response B: Incorrect. The statement is true with many of the antibodies having unexpected cross-reactivity.

Learning Response C: Incorrect. The statement is true. These are IgM antibodies which occur spontaneously.

Learning Response D: Correct. This statement is untrue. The 'natural antibodies' are low affinity IgM.

Learning Response E: Incorrect. The statement is actually true. The $CD5^+$ B cells produce natural antibodies without obvious external stimulation and presumably are mutually activated through their interactive idiotypic network.

---

393. SUBJECT AREA: Antigen drive
QUESTION: Autoantigen selection of responding B cells is indicated by:

A: Germ line configuration of the antibody
B: High affinity antibody
C: Expression of a public idiotype
D: A monoclonal antibody response
E: A response to many different autoantigens

☐ Correct Answer: *B*

Learning Response A: Incorrect. Mutation away from the germline generates antibodies, some of which are of higher affinity and will be selected by antigen in the germinal center.

Learning Response B: Correct. The mutation of B cells in the germinal center produces a range of antibody affinities, and those B cells bearing higher affinity antibody will be favorably selected for further stimulation by antigen.

Learning Response C: Incorrect. Expression of a public idiotype indicates the probable operation of an idiotypic network involving either a T-helper or an anti-idiotype directed against this common idiotype.

Learning Response D: Incorrect. The monoclonal antibody response occurs through spontaneous uncontrolled proliferation of a B-cell clone as, for example, in myeloma.

Learning Response E: Incorrect. A response to many different autoantigens could arise from polyclonal activation of lymphocytes.

394. SUBJECT AREA: T-helper bypass
QUESTION: Which of the following is *incorrect*. T-helpers can be bypassed by:

A: Failure of suppressor T cells
B: Polyclonal activation of B cells
C: Idiotypic mechanisms
D: Antigenic cross-reaction
E: T-cell recognition of carrier complexed to autoantigen

☐ Correct Answer: *A*

Learning Response A: Correct. Failure of suppressor T cells would release the T-helper for direct stimulation by antigen. This statement is therefore incorrect, since this would not be a bypass of the T-helpers.

Learning Response B: Incorrect. This statement is true because it obviates the need for T-helpers.

Learning Response C: Incorrect. Cross-reaction of exogenous antigen with an idiotypic determinant on a self-reactive lymphocyte can lead to direct stimulation of that lymphocyte without the necessity for antigen-specific T-helpers.

Learning Response D: Incorrect. This statement is true because antigenic cross-reaction at either B- or T-cell level between an exogenous antigen and a self-antigen can lead to direct lymphocyte stimulation.

Learning Response E: Incorrect. This is a true statement since it obviates the need for the T-helpers which directly recognize the autoantigen in question.

---

395. SUBJECT AREA: Regulatory bypass
QUESTION: In the NZB model of autoimmune hemolytic anemia:

      A: There are no T-cell regulatory abnormalities
      B: Disease is unaffected by neonatal thymectomy
      C: The red cell autoantibodies cause disease
      D: $CD5^+$ B cells are not involved in pathogenesis
      E: Thyroid autoantibodies are prevalent

☐ Correct Answer: *C*

Learning Response A: Incorrect. It is difficult to induce tolerance to protein antigens at high concentration in the NZB.

Learning Response B: Incorrect. The disease is exacerbated by neonatal thymectomy.

Learning Response C: Correct. Transfection with rearranged genes encoding a red cell autoantibody causes early disease in normal animals.

Learning Response D: Incorrect. Transgenic animals bearing the rearranged genes encoding pathogenic red cell autoantibody only had $CD5^+$ B cells; IP injection of red cells deleted these B cells and prevented disease.

Learning Response E: Incorrect. The model is closer to those of systemic autoimmunity and there is little overlap with organ-specific thyroid disease.

396. SUBJECT AREA: Core Revision
QUESTION: An example of a non-organ-specific (systemic) autoimmune disease is:

A: Hashimoto's thyroiditis
B: Graves' thyrotoxicosis
C: Systemic lupus erythematosus (SLE)
D: Pernicious anemia
E: Goodpasture's syndrome

☐ Correct Answer: *C*

Learning Response A: Incorrect. Hashimoto's thyroiditis involves inflammatory cell attacks specifically on the thyroid. There are organ-specific antibodies directed to thyroglobulin and the thyroid peroxidase.

Learning Response B: Incorrect. Graves' thyrotoxicosis involves stimulation of the thyroid by antibodies specific for the thyroid stimulating hormone receptor.

Learning Response C: Correct. SLE involves non-organ specific antibodies such as those against DNA and a range of other self-components which lead to production of immune complexes producing inflammation in different parts of the vascular bed, e.g., kidney, skin, brain and joints.

Learning Response D: Incorrect. Pernicious anemia involves inflammatory cell attack on the gastric mucosa with antibodies to parietal cells and intrinsic factor.

Learning Response E: Incorrect. Goodpasture's syndrome is associated with antibodies to the glomerular basement membrane of the kidney.

397. SUBJECT AREA: Core Revision
QUESTION: The NZBxW F1 hybrid provides an example of autoimmune disease that is:

A: Experimentally induced systemic
B: Spontaneous systemic
C: Experimentally induced organ-specific
D: Spontaneous organ-specific
E: None of the above

☐ Correct Answer: *B*

Learning Response A: Incorrect. An example of experimentally induced systemic autoimmune disease would be that caused by production of autoantibodies when parental T cells are injected into an F1 animal producing graft vs host disease.

Learning Response B: Correct. The animals spontaneously develop antibodies to DNA and immune complex glomerulonephritis.

Learning Response C: Incorrect. Example of experimentally induced organ-specific autoimmune disease is the experimental autoallergic encephalomyelitis induced by injection of the brain myelin basic protein in Complete Freund's adjuvant.

Learning Response D: Incorrect. An example of spontaneous organ-specific autoimmune disease is the diabetes in the NOD (non-obese diabetic) mouse. This mounts an organ-specific attack on the β cells of the pancreas and resembles the human condition of insulin-dependent diabetes in many respects.

Learning Response E: Incorrect.

---

398. SUBJECT AREA: Core Revision
QUESTION: Which factors can influence the development of autoimmune disease:

  A: Sex
  B: HLA
  C: Complement deficiency
  D: Infection
  E: All the above

☐ Correct Answer: *E*

Learning Response A: Incorrect. The statement is true but not as complete an answer as answer E.

Learning Response B: Incorrect. The statement is true but not as complete an answer as answer E.

Learning Response C: Incorrect. The statement is true but not as complete an answer as answer E.

Learning Response D: Incorrect. The statement is true but not as complete an answer as answer E.

Learning Response E: Correct.

399. SUBJECT AREA: Core revision
QUESTION: 'Natural antibodies' in the mouse are produced by:

        A: Pre-B cells
        B: CD5$^+$ B-cells
        C: CD4 cells
        D: CD8 cells
        E: NK cells

☐ Correct Answer: *B*

Learning Response A: Incorrect. Pre-B cells represent an early phase of B-cell ontogeny before the ability to secrete antibody is acquired.

Learning Response B: Correct. CD5$^+$ B cells spontaneously synthesize IgM natural antibodies initially independently of antigen stimulation, probably as a result of interidiotypic reactions. The natural antibodies are directed against common bacterial antigens and also certain autoantigens.

Learning Response C: Incorrect. CD4 cells are T cells which do not make antibody.

Learning Response D: Incorrect. CD8 cells are T cells which do not make antibody.

Learning Response E: Incorrect. NK cells do not make antibody.

400. SUBJECT AREA: Core revision
QUESTION: High affinity mutated autoantibodies imply:

        A: The recruitment of CD5$^+$ B cells
        B: Stimulation by superantigen
        C: Stimulation by clusters of autoantigens
        D: B-cell selection by autoantigen
        E: B-cell selection by anti-idiotype

☐ Correct Answer: *D*

Learning Response A: Incorrect. CD5$^+$ B cells are thymus-independent IgM producers which do not mutate to form high affinity antibodies. They do make low affinity autoantibodies of wide cross-reactivity.

Learning Response B: Incorrect. Superantigen stimulates a given Vβ family independently of antigen. They are T cells.

Learning Response C: Incorrect. High affinity autoantibody implies selection by antigen but gives no evidence that they are caused by a cluster of autoantigens unless they form a pattern of reactivity against a given cluster of autoantigens. If such a cluster is connected by anatomical location, this is an indication of antigen drive of the autoimmune response.

Learning Response D: Correct. B cells which mutate in the germinal centers to form higher affinity surface antibodies will be preferentially selected by autoantigen.

Learning Response E: Incorrect. Anti-idiotypes cannot provide the selection process in the germinal center for higher affinity mutated autoantibodies that the antigen itself does.

---

401. SUBJECT AREA: Core revision
QUESTION: Which of the following responses is *incorrect*. Autoimmunity can arise when:

- A: Exogenous antigens cross-react with self-antigen
- B: Exogenous antigens cross-react with self-idiotypes
- C: B cells are stimulated with polyclonal activators
- D: T suppressors are stimulated
- E: Cytokine imbalance occurs

☐ Correct Answer: *D*

Learning Response A: Incorrect. The statement is true. Cross-reaction with a B-cell epitope but providing a new helper T epitope will induce autoimmunity. So will cross-reaction with a self–T-cell epitope recognized by cryptic T cells which have not been tolerized in the thymus.

Learning Response B: Incorrect. The statement is true. Immune response to an exogenous antigen which cross-reacts with an idiotype on a self-reactive B or T cell will stimulate autoimmunity.

Learning Response C: Incorrect. The statement is true. Polyclonal activators will stimulate most T cells including some which are self-reactive but not tolerized.

Learning Response D: Correct. The statement is untrue because T suppressors would presumably suppress. However one could conceive an unlikely scenario in which T-suppressors suppressed suppressors of autoimmunity. No evidence for this exists at the moment.

Learning Response E: Incorrect. The statement is true. Insertion of an interferon-γ gene into the islet cell stimulates autoimmunity to the pancreas.

---

402. SUBJECT AREA: Pathogenic effects of humoral autoantibody
QUESTION: The antiphospholipid syndrome is associated with:

      A: Infertility
      B: Severe anemia
      C: Wegener's granulomatosis
      D: Raised platelet levels
      E: Recurrent fetal loss

☐ Correct Answer: *E*

Learning Response A: Incorrect. Although some autoimmune phenomena can lead to infertility, this is not the case in the antiphospholipid syndrome.

Learning Response B: Incorrect. Autoimmune hemolytic anemia is an autoimmune disease where autoantibodies to erythrocytes causes severe anemia.

Learning Response C: Incorrect. Wegener's granulomatosis is characterized by autoantibodies to proteinase III, an intracellular antigen associated with the primary granules of polymorphs which translocates to the cell surface following cytokine-mediated activation of the cell, a location which can then be the target for an antibody-mediated immune attack.

Learning Response D: Incorrect. In fact in the antiphospholipid syndrome there are reduced levels of platelets, i.e., thrombocytopenia.

Learning Response E: Correct. Recurrent fetal loss is characteristic of the antiphospholipid syndrome. In the experimental situation, passive transfer of cardiolipin antibodies into mice also results in recurrent fetal loss.

---

403. SUBJECT AREA: Pathogenic effects of humoral autoantibody
QUESTION: An alternative name for thyrotoxicosis is:

      A: Hashimoto's disease
      B: Primary myxedema
      C: Graves' disease

D: Exophthalmos
E: Goiter

☐ Correct Answer: *C*

Learning Response A: Incorrect. Like thyrotoxicosis, Hashimoto's disease results from an autoimmune reaction with the thyroid, but in this case can lead to hypothyroidism (due to destruction of the gland) rather than the hyperthyroidism associated with thyrotoxicosis.

Learning Response B: Incorrect. Another thyroid autoimmune disorder with mononuclear inflammatory cell attack on the gland as in Hashimoto's disease, but with inevitable hypothyroidism due to blocking antibodies to the TSH receptor.

Learning Response C: Correct. A third name sometimes given to this disease is Basedow's disease. There is a hyperthyroidism due to stimulating autoantibodies to the TSH receptor which continuously mimic the effect of TSH but which are not subject to the feedback mechanisms which lower the level of TSH once sufficient thyroid hormone has been produced.

Learning Response D: Incorrect. Exophthalmos is often associated with thyrotoxicosis, but specifically refers to the marked hypertrophy of the extra-occular muscles. It may be due to antibodies directed to a 64 kDa membrane protein present on both eye muscle and thyroid.

Learning Response E: Incorrect. Goiter simply refers to an enlarged thyroid which may be due to thyroid autoimmune disease but can also be caused by iodine deficiency or carcinoma.

404. SUBJECT AREA: Pathogenic effects of humoral autoantibody
QUESTION: Neonatal myasthenia gravis is thought to be caused by:

A: An inherited genetic defect
B: Transplacental transfer of maternal IgG against the TSH receptor
C: Anti-idiotype to maternal IgG
D: Transplacental transfer of maternal IgG against the acetylcholine receptor
E: Maternal T cells transferred across the placenta

☐ Correct Answer: *D*

Learning Response A: Incorrect. Although there are inherited genetic contributions towards the development of autoimmune diseases, these diseases are multifactorial in nature and not a straighforward gene defect in the way that, say, Duchenne muscular dystrophy is.

Learning Response B: Incorrect. Transplacental transfer of maternal IgG anti-thyroid stimulating hormone (TSH) receptor does cause a neonatal autoimmune syndrome, but this is neonatal thyrotoxicosis in the offspring of mothers with Graves' disease.

Learning Response C: Incorrect. Anti-idiotypes to maternal anti-acetylcholine receptor may occur in the babies of mothers with myasthenia gravis, but these are thought to be protective against neonatal myasthenia gravis by blocking the effects of the autoantibody.

Learning Response D: Correct. Transient neonatal autoimmune diseases are seen due to the transplacental transfer of maternal IgG autoantibodies. The disease will be of the same type as seen in the mother because the autoantibodies will determine the target organ specificity. The neonatal disease resolves after a few weeks as the maternal IgG is catabolized.

Learning Response E: Incorrect. Lymphocytes are not transferred across the placenta. With respect to antibodies, only IgG is transferred because there is a specific transport mechanism which only recognizes this class of antibody.

405. SUBJECT AREA: Pathogenic effects of humoral autoantibody
QUESTION: In celiac disease there is T-cell sensitivity to:

A: Vitamin B_{12}
B: Gluten
C: β-adrenergic receptors
D: Gastric H^+K^+ dependent ATPase
E: Myelin basic protein

☐ Correct Answer: *B*

Learning Response A: Incorrect. Autoantibodies to intrinsic factor inhibit vitamin B_{12} uptake in pernicious anemia.

Learning Response B: Correct. The normally acquired tolerance to the dietary protein wheat gluten breaks down in celiac disease. Because gluten binds strongly to the extracellular matrix protein endomyceum, this may lead to an autoimmune attack on the gut by endomyceum-specific IgA antibodies. These may be triggered by 'piggy-back' presentation of gluten to gluten-specific T cells by the endomyceum-specific B cells.

Learning Response C: Incorrect. Blocking antibodies to β-adrenergic receptors may represent one of the factors which alter the baseline sensitivity of mast cells in patients with atopic allergy.

Learning Response D: Incorrect. Patients with pernicious anemia have inhibitory antibodies which bind to this gastric proton pump leading to hypochlorohydria, a lack of acid production in the stomach.

Learning Response E: Incorrect. T cells specific for MBP are found in patients with multiple sclerosis and induction of an MBP-specific T-cell response in rodents leads to experimental autoimmune encephalomyelitis (EAE), a demyelinating disease with features similar to human multiple sclerosis.

---

406. SUBJECT AREA: Pathogenic effects of humoral autoantibody
QUESTION: Glomerulonephritis associated with pulmonary hemorrhage is referred to as:

> *A:* Pemphigus vulgaris
> *B:* Goodpasture's syndrome
> *C:* Systemic lupus erythematosus
> *D:* Lambert-Eaton syndrome
> *E:* Wegener's granulomatosis

☐ Correct Answer: *B*

Learning Response A: Incorrect. Pemphigus vulgaris is an autoimmune disease affecting the skin in which autoantibodies are present against a member of the cadherin adhesion molecule family found on stratified squamous epithelium.

Learning Response B: Correct. The association is due to autoantibodies to glomerular basement membrane which cross-react with alveolar basement membrane.

Learning Response C: Incorrect. Patients with SLE often have an immune-complex mediated glomerulonephritis, but not usually pulmonary hemorrhage, although many do have shortness of breath, pleurisy and pleural effusions.

Learning Response D: Incorrect. Lambert-Eaton syndrome involves neuromuscular defects associated with antibodies to pre-synaptic calcium channels.

Learning Response E: Incorrect. Wegener's granulomatosis is characterized by anti-neutrophil cytoplasmic antibodies (cANCA) specific for proteinase III.

---

407. SUBJECT AREA: Pathogenic effects of complexes with autoantigens
QUESTION: A spontaneous model of systemic lupus erythematosus is the:

- *A:* Balb/c mouse
- *B:* MRL-*lpr/lpr* mouse
- *C:* SJL mouse
- *D:* Obese strain chicken
- *E:* SCID mouse

☐ Correct Answer: *B*

Learning Response A: Incorrect. Balb/c is a relatively normal inbred strain of mouse which does not usually develop autoimmune disease spontaneously.

Learning Response B: Correct. The MRL strain of mouse homozygous for the lymphoproliferative gene *lpr* develops an immune-complex mediated glomerular nephritis as seen in some patients with SLE. MRL strain mice lacking the *lpr* gene (MRL/+) develop a less severe, later onset, form of the disease.

Learning Response C: Incorrect. The SJL mouse does not develop spontaneous autoimmune disease but appears unable to regulate certain immune responses, perhaps due to a defect in suppressor pathways. For example, if normal mice are injected with rat erythrocytes, they exhibit a transient autoimmune hemolytic anemia (AHA) due to the production of erythrocyte antibodies which cross-react with the mouse's own erythrocytes. In SJL mice this normally transient AHA is not corrected and proves fatal.

Learning Response D: Incorrect. The obese strain chicken does develop a spontaneous autoimmune disease, but it is an organ-specific thyroid autoimmunity similar to Hashimoto's disease rather than the non-organ specific SLE.

Learning Response E: Incorrect. The SCID mouse is profoundly immunodeficient, lacking both mature T and B cells.

---

408. SUBJECT AREA: Pathogenic effects of complexes with autoantigens
QUESTION: In rheumatoid arthritis the non-lymphoid synovial tissue shows aberrant expression of:

A: Immunoglobulin genes
B: T-cell receptor genes
C: MHC class I
D: MHC class II
E: MHC class III

☐ Correct Answer: *D*

Learning Response A: Incorrect. Immunoglobulin genes are only expressed by B lymphocytes. Note, however, that in RA there is a large amount of antibody produced by B cells within the inflamed synovium.

Learning Response B: Incorrect. T-cell receptor genes are only expressed by T lymphocytes. Note, however, that in RA there is T-cell proliferation within the inflamed synovium.

Learning Response C: Incorrect. Like most nucleated cells in the body, synovial tissue normally expresses MHC class I molecules, although the level of expression is often increased in RA.

Learning Response D: Correct. MHC class II is normally only expressed by professional antigen-presenting cells such as dendritic cells, B cells and activated macrophages. However, in a number of autoimmune diseases, including RA, the affected tissue shows aberrant expression of MHC class II, probably in response to increased levels of cytokines such as IFNγ and TNFα.

Learning Response E: Incorrect. MHC class III is a term sometimes used to denote the non-antigen-presenting molecules encoded within the MHC gene locus. These include TNFα, TNFβ, and the complement components C2 and C4.

409. SUBJECT AREA: Core revision
QUESTION: Rheumatoid factors are:

A: DNA–anti-DNA immune complexes
B: Autoantibodies to IgM
C: Autoantibodies to complement components
D: Autoantibodies to IgG
E: Any factor predisposing to rheumatoid arthritis

☐ Correct Answer: *D*

Learning Response A: Incorrect. DNA–anti-DNA immune complexes are often found in patients with systemic lupus erythematosus (SLE).

Learning Response B: Incorrect. The rheumatoid factors themselves can be IgM, IgG or IgA, but they are not autoantibodies to IgM.

Learning Response C: Incorrect. Autoantibodies to complement components are called immunoconglutinins. Rheumatoid factor may fix complement once it has bound to its specific antigen.

Learning Response D: Correct. Autoantibodies to IgG Fc regions may be of the IgG, IgM or IgA class. Although found in patients with rheumatoid arthritis, these rheumatoid factors are also frequently seen in many other conditions and therefore are not by themselves diagnostic for RA.

Learning Response E: Incorrect. Like other autoimmune diseases, RA is thought to be multifactorial in nature, but the term rheumatoid factor is reserved for a specific type of autoantibody.

---

410. SUBJECT AREA: Pathogenic effects of complexes with autoantigens
QUESTION: IgG in patients with rheumatoid arthritis has abnormal:

- *A:* Glycosylation
- *B:* Disulfide bonds
- *C:* Light chain sequence
- *D:* Hinge regions
- *E:* Valency

☐ Correct Answer: *A*

Learning Response A: Correct. A decrease in the total amount of galactose is seen on the N-linked oligosaccharide of the IgG Fc.

Learning Response B: Incorrect. The disulfide bonds are the same as in the IgG from normal individuals, i.e., one intra-chain disulfide-bond per domain, one disulfide bond linking each light chain to the adjacent heavy chain, and a varying number of inter-heavy chain disulfide bonds depending on the IgG subclass.

Learning Response C: Incorrect. The light chain sequences are not abnormal in rheumatoid arthritis.

Learning Response D: Incorrect. The hinge region provides molecular flexibility to the antibody molecule and is normal in rheumatoid arthritis.

Learning Response E: Incorrect. IgG from patients with RA has the normal two arm structure each with an identical antigen-binding specificity.

---

411. SUBJECT AREA: Core revision
QUESTION: In rheumatoid arthritis, the outgrowth of synovial lining cells which produces erosions in the underlying cartilage and bone is called:

   A: Opsonin
   B: Proteoglycan
   C: Pannus
   D: The Arthus reaction
   E: Frustrated phagocytosis

☐ Correct Answer: *C*

Learning Response A: Incorrect. An opsonin is a molecule such as antibody or complement which by coating an antigen makes it more readily phagocytosed. This will usually be due to binding to Fc receptors and/or complement receptors on the phagocyte.

Learning Response B: Incorrect. Proteoglycans form part of the articular cartilage which is subject to enzymatic attack in RA.

Learning Response C: Correct. The term pannus refers to the activated synovial cells which grow out as a malign cover over the cartilage. They produce erosions in the underlying cartilage and bone through the release of IL-1, IL-6, TNFα, PGE$_2$, collagenase, neutral proteinase and reactive oxygen intermediates.

Learning Response D: Incorrect. The Arthus reaction leads to an influx of polymorphs into the synovial cavity.

Learning Response E: Incorrect. The term frustrated phagocytosis is used to denote a situation in which a phagocyte is unable to internalize an antigen which it has been triggered by, e.g., because it is part of a large insoluble surface such as articular cartilage.

---

412. SUBJECT AREA: T-cell mediated hypersensitivity in autoimmune diseases
QUESTION: Arthritis can be induced in rats by injection of:

   A: Pooled normal rat IgG
   B: Freund's incomplete adjuvant

C: Freund's complete adjuvant
D: A T-cell clone specific for thyroglobulin
E: α_2-macroglobulin

☐ Correct Answer: C

Learning Response A: Incorrect. Although rheumatoid arthritis is associated with the presence of rheumatoid factor, i.e., autoantibodies to the Fc portion of IgG, injection of pooled normal rat IgG induces neither rheumatoid factor nor arthritis.

Learning Response B: Incorrect. Freund's incomplete adjuvant, a water in oil emulsion that is often used as an adjuvant, does not induce arthritis if injected alone into rats.

Learning Response C: Correct. The critical component in the induction of adjuvant arthritis is the mycobacteria in the Freund's complete adjuvant. The microorganisms contain an hsp60 which shares an amino acid sequence with cartilage proteoglycan and which is recognized by pathogenic T cells.

Learning Response D: Incorrect. Thyroglobulin is an autoantigen recognized in an organ-specific animal model of autoimmunity, experimental autoimmune thyroiditis (EAT). Some T-cell clones are able to transfer the disease.

Learning Response E: Incorrect. α_2-macroglobulin is an enzyme inhibitor.

413. SUBJECT AREA: T-cell mediated hypersensitivity in autoimmune diseases
QUESTION: The inflammatory infiltrate in autoimmune thyroiditis comprises mostly:

A: Phagocytic cells
B: Polymorphonuclear leukocytes
C: Lymphocytes
D: Mast cells
E: Eosinophils

☐ Correct Answer: C

Learning Response A: Incorrect. Although both macrophages and neutrophils are found infiltrating the thyroid in autoimmune thyroiditis, they do not form the dominant cell population.

Learning Response B: Incorrect. Some polymorphs are found as these cells are generally present at sites of inflammation, but they are not the dominant cell type in this case.

Learning Response C: Correct. Lymphocytes constitute the bulk of the infiltrate, with the dominant population being CD4$^+$ T cells, although CD8$^+$ T cells and B cells are also present. Macrophages constitute a significant minor population.

Learning Response D: Incorrect. Few if any mast cells are found in the inflammatory infiltrate in autoimmune thyroiditis. Such cells are normally found at the sites of IgE-mediated allergic reactions.

Learning Response E: Incorrect. The occasional eosinophil is present and may partake in ADCC-type reactions but they are not the dominant cell type.

---

414. SUBJECT AREA: T-cell mediated hypersensitivity in autoimmune diseases
QUESTION: In insulin-dependent diabetes mellitus, the target of the autoimmune attack is:

A: All of the cells in the islets of Langerhans
B: The β cells in the islets of Langerhans
C: The somatostatin-producing cells in the islets of Langerhans
D: The glucagon-producing cells in the islets of Langerhans
E: Cells throughout the body which have an insulin receptor

☐ Correct Answer: *B*

Learning Response A: Incorrect. The attack is on cells in the islets of Langerhans but is selective for only one particular type of cell.

Learning Response B: Correct. It is antigens associated with the insulin-producing β cells which are the target of the autoimmune attack, although the precise antigens involved are still under investigation; glutamic acid decarboxylase (GAD) is probably an important autoantigen in this disease.

Learning Response C: Incorrect. The somatostatin-producing cells in the islets of Langerhans do not possess the antigens that are the targets of the autoimmune attack.

Learning Response D: Incorrect. The glucagon-producing cells in the islets of Langerhans do not possess the antigens that are the targets of the autoimmune attack.

Learning Response E: Incorrect. The insulin receptor is not a major target of the autoimmune attack which is restricted to the pancreas, i.e., insulin-dependent diabetes mellitus (IDDM) is an organ-specific autoimmune disease.

415. SUBJECT AREA: Core revision
QUESTION: An animal model of insulin-dependent diabetes mellitus is the:

- *A:* Obese strain chicken
- *B:* (NZB x NZW) F_1 mouse
- *C:* BXSB mouse
- *D:* Brown Norway rat
- *E:* NOD mouse

☐ Correct Answer: *E*

Learning Response A: Incorrect. The Obese strain chicken is a spontaneous animal model for human autoimmune thyroiditis (Hashimoto's disease).

Learning Response B: Incorrect. The (NZB x NZW) F_1 mouse is an animal model for systemic lupus erythematosus (SLE). The parental NZB strain develops an autoimmune hemolytic anemia.

Learning Response C: Incorrect. The BXSB mouse is an animal model for systemic lupus erythematosus (SLE).

Learning Response D: Incorrect. When the Brown Norway rat is injected with mercuric chloride it develops an anti-glomerular basement membrane-associated glomerulonephritis. It is therefore used as an animal model of Goodpasture's syndrome.

Learning Response E: Correct. The non-obese diabetic (NOD) mouse is a spontaneous animal model of insulin-dependent diabetes mellitus. T cells from diseased NOD mice can produce typical pancreatic lesions when transferred into young mice of the same strain.

416. SUBJECT AREA: T-cell mediated hypersensitivity in autoimmune diseases
QUESTION: An animal model for multiple sclerosis is:

- *A:* EAT
- *B:* EAE
- *C:* NOD mouse

D: Nude mouse
E: MRL-*lpr/lpr* mouse

☐ Correct Answer: *B*

Learning Response A: Incorrect. Experimental autoimmune thyroiditis (EAT) is an animal model for human autoimmune thyroiditis (Hashimoto's disease). It is conventionally produced by injection of thyroglobulin in complete Freund's adjuvant.

Learning Response B: Correct. Experimental autoimmune encephalomyelitis (EAE) is produced by injection of myelin basic protein (MBP) in complete Freund's adjuvant. This leads to a demyelinating disease with resultant motor paralysis, similar to human multiple sclerosis.

Learning Response C: Incorrect. The NOD mouse develops a spontaneous autoimmune disease which parallels human insulin-dependent diabetes mellitus (IDDM).

Learning Response D: Incorrect. Nude mice are congenitally athymic, as are human subjects with DiGeorge syndrome. This leads to a profound T-cell deficiency.

Learning Response E: Incorrect. MRL strain mice homozygous for the *lpr* (lymphoproliferative) gene develop a severe SLE-like disease.

417. SUBJECT AREA: Treatment of autoimmune disorders
QUESTION: Pernicious anemia can be treated with:

A: Thyroxine
B: Insulin
C: Vitamin B_{12}
D: Thymectomy
E: Acetylcholinesterase inhibitors

☐ Correct Answer: *C*

Learning Response A: Incorrect. Thyroxine is a thyroid hormone (tetraiodothyronine, T4) which is given to patients with primary myxedema and Hashimoto's disease (both resulting from a destructive autoimmune thyroiditis) to compensate for the hypothyroidism and also in the latter case, to inhibit goiter formation by the excessive TSH production. The primary myxedema patients are not goitrous because they have blocking antibodies to the TSH receptor.

Learning Response B: Incorrect. Insulin is given to patients with insulin-dependent diabetes mellitus (IDDM) to compensate for the destruction of the insulin-producing β cells in the islets of Langerhans in the pancreas.

Learning Response C: Correct. In pernicious anemia there are autoantibodies to intrinsic factor (IF) in the stomach which prevent the uptake of the intrinsic factor-vitamin B_{12} complex by blocking the binding of IF to its receptor, or by blocking the binding of B_{12} to IF. Injections of vitamin B_{12} overcome this inability to transport vitamin B_{12} across the gut wall.

Learning Response D: Incorrect. Thymectomy has no effect on pernicious anemia but is of benefit in the treatment of myasthenia gravis, possibly because the thymus contains acetylcholine receptors in a particularly immunogenic form.

Learning Response E: Incorrect. Acetylcholinesterase inhibitors are commonly used for the long term treatment of myasthenia gravis.

418. SUBJECT AREA: Treatment of autoimmune disorders
QUESTION: A therapeutic approach in rheumatoid arthritis might be to:

  A: Stimulate TNFα production
  B: Inhibit TNFα activity
  C: Reduce TGFβ secretion
  D: Administer silver salts
  E: Use prostaglandin

☐ Correct Answer: *B*

Learning Response A: Incorrect. TNFα is a pro-inflammatory cytokine and therefore to stimulate its production would be likely to exacerbate the disease.

Learning Response B: Correct. TNFα is a pro-inflammatory cytokine and treatment of patients with RA using a chimeric human-mouse antibody to TNFα has been shown to lead to a reduction in severity of various disease parameters.

Learning Response C: Incorrect. TGFβ is a suppressive cytokine and one might therefore want to enhance its secretion at the site of the autoimmune attack, rather than reduce it.

Learning Response D: Incorrect. Gold, not silver, salts are effective in the treatment of RA, although their mode of action is not understood.

Learning Response E: Incorrect. Prostaglandin secretion by macrophages may well contribute toward the damage in RA joints, and one gives prostaglandin inhibitors, not prostaglandin, to these patients.

419. SUBJECT AREA: Treatment of autoimmune disorders
QUESTION: Animals have been protected against EAE by immunization with:

- *A:* T-cell receptor Vα peptide
- *B:* Pooled normal immunoglobulin
- *C:* Myelin basic protein in complete Freund's adjuvant
- *D:* T-cell receptor Vβ peptide
- *E:* An encephalitogenic peptide

☐ Correct Answer: *D*

Learning Response A: Incorrect. Immunization with an attenuated T-cell clone specific for myelin basic protein can protect against the induction of EAE.

Learning Response B: Incorrect. Interestingly, intravenous immunoglobulin pooled from a large number of normal donors leads to a clinical improvement in a number of autoimmune conditions in man. This may be due to antiidiotypes in the pooled Ig 'resetting' an imbalanced idiotype network in the patients but the mechanisms are poorly understood.

Learning Response C: Incorrect. Myelin basic protein in complete Freund's adjuvant is used to induce EAE, not protect against its induction.

Learning Response D: Correct. A synthetic peptide based on the Vβ sequence from an encephalitogenic T-cell clone induces suppressive $CD8^+$ T cells specific for this peptide presented by MHC class I molecules.

Learning Response E: Incorrect. The term encephalitogenic refers to a molecule or cell that is able to induce encephalomyelitis, not protect against its induction.

420. SUBJECT AREA: Treatment of autoimmune disorders
QUESTION: Immune defenses in the gut have evolved mechanisms which restrict the activation of:

A: T_{h1} cells
B: T_{h2} cells
C: B cells
D: Cytotoxic T lymphocytes
E: Mast cells

☐ Correct Answer: *A*

Learning Response A: Correct. Enterocytes are especially vulnerable to damage by the T_{h1}-produced cytokines IFNγ and TNF. Thus, T_{h2} cells are preferentially stimulated and the TGFβ they release inhibits the activation of T_{h1} cells.

Learning Response B: Incorrect. Quite the opposite. T_{h2} cells are preferentially stimulated in the gut. These are producers of TGFβ, which is able to suppress the activity of the IFNγ and TNF-producing T_{h1} cells.

Learning Response C: Incorrect. B cells, particularly those secreting antibodies of the IgA class, are active in the gut as one of the first line defences against infection.

Learning Response D: Incorrect. CTL are able to function in the gut, although T cells bearing the γδ form of the T-cell receptor may be particularly important in patrolling this anatomical location.

Learning Response E: Incorrect. Mast cells provide an important protective mechanism when triggered to release vasoactive amines by IgE antibodies specific for gut parasites such as nematodes.

421. SUBJECT AREA: Core revision
QUESTION: Thyrocytes expressing MHC class II in autoimmune thyroid disease are direct targets for locally activated T cells specific for:

A: PMN proteinase III
B: Acetylcholine receptor
C: Cardiolipin/$β_2$-glycoprotein 1 complex
D: A peroxidase enzyme
E: Presynaptic calcium channels

☐ Correct Answer: *D*

Learning Response A: Incorrect. The proteinase III of polymorphonuclear (PMN) leukocytes is implicated in the PMN-induced endothelial injury seen in Wegener's granulomatosis.

Learning Response B: Incorrect. The acetylcholine receptor is the major autoantigen in myasthenia gravis.

Learning Response C: Incorrect. Autoantibodies to the cardiolipin/β_2-glycoprotein 1 complex are responsible for the recurrent thromboembotic phenomena seen in the anti-phospholipid syndrome.

Learning Response D: Correct. The expression of MHC class II molecules on the thyrocytes of patients with autoimmune thyroiditis make these cells targets for thyroid peroxidase-specific T cells.

Learning Response E: Incorrect. Antibodies to the pre-synaptic calcium channels are thought to be responsible for the neuromuscular defect in Lambert-Eaton syndrome.

---

422. SUBJECT AREA: Core revision

QUESTION: A difference between organ-specific and nonorgan-specific autoimmune disorders is that:

- *A:* Only in organ-specific autoimmune disorders is there a greater incidence in women
- *B:* Associations with HLA are only seen in nonorgan-specific autoimmunity
- *C:* Circulating autoantibodies react with normal body components only in organ-specific autoimmune disorders
- *D:* It is only in organ-specific autoimmune disorders that autoantibody tests are of diagnostic value
- *E:* Only in organ-specific autoimmune diseases is therapy aimed at controlling metabolic defects

☐ Correct Answer: *E*

Learning Response A: Incorrect. There is a general trend for autoimmune disease to occur far more frequently in women than in men. This is seen in both organ-specific (e.g., in Graves' thyrotoxicosis the female:male incidence is 7:1) and nonorgan-specific (e.g., SLE 10:1) autoimmune disorders.

Learning Response B: Incorrect. Association of HLA with autoimmune disease is seen in both organ-specific (e.g., in insulin-dependent diabetes mellitus DR3/4 heterozygotes carry a relative risk of 14.3) and nonorgan-specific (e.g., in rheumatoid arthritis DR4 carries a relative risk of 5.8) diseases.

Learning Response C: Incorrect. Circulating autoantibodies react with normal body components in both organ-specific and nonorgan-specific autoimmune diseases.

Learning Response D: Incorrect. In myasthenia gravis (an organ-specific autoimmune disease) >80% of patients have readily detectable autoantibodies to the acetylcholine receptor. Autoantibodies to double-stranded DNA are characteristic of the nonorgan-specific autoimmune disease SLE.

Learning Response E: Correct. In many organ-specific autoimmune diseases metabolic control provides an adequate means of correcting the deficit produced by organ destruction. Thus, thyroxine replacement is given in primary myxedema, insulin in insulin-dependent diabetes mellitus, vitamin B_{12} in pernicious anemia, and so forth. In nonorgan-specific autoimmune diseases the therapy is aimed at inhibiting inflammation and antibody synthesis.

INDEX

Numbers after index entries represent question numbers.

ABO, cross-matching for MHC and, 362
Abzyme, 118
Accessory molecule, 66
Acetylcholinesterase inhibitor, 417
Acetylcholine receptor, 341, 386, 421
    transplacental transfer of maternal IgG against, 404
Acidic dye, 14
Acquired immunity, 30, 37
    adoptive transfer and, 33
Acquired immunodeficiency syndrome (AIDS), 367
    AZT and, 316
    CD4 T-cell depletion and, 322
    diagnosis of, 314
    HIV and, 310–312, 315
    lesions of, 313
Acquired memory, 31–33, 36, 37
Acute inflammation, 2, 9, 20
    initiation of, 18
Acute myeloid leukemia (AML), 369
Acute phase protein(s), 11, 19
    cytokines mediate release of, 189
Adaptive immune response
    major factor in regulation of, 194
    negative feedback on, 196
    T cells and, 25
Addison's disease, 364, 389
Adenoid, 133
Adhesion, 149
Adhesion molecule
    CD44 and, 372
    upregulation of, 251, 276
Adjuvant, 107
Adoptive transfer of acquired immune responsiveness, 33
Adrenal, Addison's disease of, 389
Afferent lymphatics, 137
Affinity, 88, 105, 106
Affinity chromatography, 120
African children, 376
Ag_2Ab_1 immune complex, 102
Agar, 111, 113
Agglutination test, 107
Agranulocytosis, 332
Agretope, 301
Alimentary tract, 148
Alkaline phosphatase, 109, 123
Allelic exclusion, 237, 248
Allelic polymorphism, 46, 81
Allergen(s), 108
    cloning of, 328
Allergic bronchopulmonary aspergillosis, 104
Allergy, 108, 349
    atopic, 405
Allogeneic graft, 343–345
    immunosuppression and, 363
    rejection of, 362
    second, very rapid response for, 359
Allotype, 46, 324
α chain, 68, 149, 150, 191
α-fetoprotein, 385
α-helix, 78
αα homodimer, T-cell receptor, 235
αβ heterodimer, 235
    IL-2 receptor, 177
αβ T cell, fetal, 236
αβ T cell receptor gene, 240
Alternative complement pathway, 6, 7, 17, 21, 24
    C3 convertase, 304
Alternative (salvage) pathway for DNA synthesis, 117
Alternative splicing, 65, 186
Aluminum hydroxide, 296
Amino acid, 66
    homogenous structure of, 58
    nonadjacent, 85
Aminopterin, 117
Ammonium sulfate, 103
Amylase of saliva, 1
Amyloid A (AA) protein, 380
Anaphylatoxin, 8, 17, 21, 24, 39
Anaphylaxis, 26, 324, 326
    passive cutaneous, 325
    in skin, 325
Anemia, severe, 402
Anergy, 156, 324
Animal(s)
    dander of, 328
    F1 (A × B), 347
    primed, 136
    protection of, against EAE, 419
    thymectomized, 231
Animal model
    of immunodeficiency, 375
    of insulin-dependent diabetes mellitus, 415
    for multiple sclerosis, 416
    for SLE, 415
Ankylosing spondylitis, 364
Antibacterial action of C-reactive protein, 20
Antibacterial antibody, 52
Antibiotic(s), 1
    colicins and, 7
    peptide, 5

Antibody(ies), 5, 21, 23, 39, 94, 259
  activation of complement by constant
      region of, 22
  in agar, 111
  antigen-binding arms of, 22
  binding of antigen and, 86
  binding strength of antigen for, 88, 95
  bivalent nature of, 102
  cell-surface and secreted versions of, 65
  cellular basis of production of, 27, 28, 34
  coating of cell with, 121
  detection of, 104
      in serum following primary contact with
          antigen, 28
  enzyme activity of, 118
  estimation of, 101, 102, 105, 107
      RAST measurements and, 108
      surface plasmon resonance and, 110
  high affinity, 184, 393
  high responses of: MHC class II genes and,
      222
      for (TG)-A-L antigen, 210
  high titer, 209
  hypersensitivity and, 339
  of identical specificity to that on surface of
      parent B cell, 27
  against individual's own body components, 30
  labeling of, with horseradish peroxidase, 109
  long-term production of, 142
  loss of binding power for, 85
  lysis by, 289
  making of, to order, 117, 119
  mediation of effector functions of, 22
  natural, 52, 202, 217, 392
      in mouse, 399
  neutralizing: target for, 315
      toxins and, 261
  preformed, 361
  protective, against infectious agents, 32
  protein vaccines and, 300
  purification of, by affinity chromatography,
      120
  regulatory idiotypes on, 206
  serum, 338
  side-chain theory of production of, 34
  specificity of, 183
      for different epitopes on same antigen, 205
      high affinity B-cell clones and, 185
  synthesis of, 187
  T-cell help for production of, 165
  variable region of, 283
Antibody-containing gel, 113
Antibody-dependent cell-mediated cytotoxicity
    (ADCC), 37, 330, 333
Antibody feedback control, 196
Antibody-producing cells, 25, 138
  enumeration of, 127
Antibody titer, 101
Anti-cardiolipin, 388

Anti-CD3, 349
Anti-CD4, 346, 362
Anti-CD4/8 treatment, 351
Anti-CD33, 383
Anti-DNA, 381, 390
Antigen(s), 21, 23, 84, 85, 94, 199
  in agar, 111
  B-cell surface receptor for, 64-66
  β-turn loop for binding of, 47
  binding of, 22, 66, 86-88
      by Fab fragment, 42, 62
  binding strength of antibody for, 95, 105, 106
  in blood, 134
  carbohydrate, 96
  for cell surface immunoglobulin on virgin
      B cell, 67
  clonal selection and, 26
  concentration of, adaptive immune response
      and, 194
  defective presentation of, 313
  depletion of, 136
  erogenous, 401
  extreme excess of, 102
  foreign, major long-term source of, 193
  gene cluster contribution to binding of, 44
  handling of: Langerhans' cells and, 144
      macrophages and, 145
  identification and measurement of: Ouchter-
      lony double diffusion method and, 111
      pepscan technique and, 116
      SDS-PAGE and, 115
      single radial immunodiffusion and, 113
      spur in Ouchterlony test and, 112
      Western blots and, 114
  labeling of Ig of, with horseradish peroxidase, 109
  level of, 217
  localization of, in tissues, 130
  low amounts of, 184
  in MHC class I groove, 98
  native, 89, 96
  primary contact with, detection of antibodies
      in serum and, 28
  processing of, 145
  purification of, by affinity chromatography,
      120
  recall, 37
  recurrent stimulation with, 192
  same, antibodies specific for different
      epitopes on, 205
  self, 247
  sequestering of, from immune system, 143
  specificity of, 30, 37
  surface Ig receptors for, 168
  T-cell receptor for, 68
  T-cell surface receptor for, 70–72
  thymus-dependent, 172
  transplantation, 345, 371
  tumor, 373
  (*See also* Specific type of antigen)

Antigen-binding arm of antibody molecule, 22
Antigen-binding single chain Fv, 286
Antigen drive, 393
Antigen-presenting cell, 92, 145, 169, 201
 antigen moiety on, 89
 MHC class II molecules on, 82, 154
 professional, 157
Antigen receptor, 25, 201, 234
 number of variable regions of, 74
Antigen recognition (signal), 372
 complementarity determining regions and, 43
 generation of diversity for, 74, 75
 by T cells, 165, 210
 transduction of, 73
Antigen shift, 268, 280
Antigen-specific B cells, purification of, 129
Antigen-specific T suppression, 197
 inhibition of, 198
Antigenic competition, 195
Anti-glomerular basement membrane (anti-GBM), 388
Anti-HLA-DQ, addition of, for lepromatous leprosy patients, 198
Anti-idiotype, 205, 207, 221, 302, 373, 393, 400
 internal image monoclonal, 208
Anti-IL-5, 349
Anti-immunoglobulin, 103, 123
 magnetic beads coated with, 121
Anti-immunoglobulin G (anti-IgG), 381, 387
Antimicrobicidal agent, 4
Anti-mitochondrial antibody, 388
Anti-neutrophil cytoplasmic antibody (ANCA), 388, 406
Anti-nuclear antibody, 387
Anti-parallel β-pleated sheet structure, 47
Anti-parietal cell, 387
Antiphospholipid syndrome, 388, 402, 421
Anti-rhesus D prophylaxis, 196
Antiserum, 101, 112, 113, 221
Anti-SS-A(Ro), 388
Anti-SS-B(La), 388
Anti-thyroglobulin, 386
Anti-thyroid peroxidase, 386, 387
Antitoxin, 5
Anti-TSH receptor, 387
Antiviral effect, 19
Apoptosis, 125, 139
 increased susceptibility for, 313
Arteriole, dilation of, 9
Arthritis, induction of, in rats, 412
Arthus reaction, 334, 411
Aspergillus precipitin, 104
Association (constant), 105, 110
 of Ag/Ab equilibrium, 88
Atopic allergy, 405
Autoallergic attack on brain, 390
Autoantibody(ies), 30, 243, 341, 381, 386
 circulating, 422
 cross-reacting, 142
 high affinity, 202
 high affinity mutated, 400
 for IgG, 409
 in mixed connective tissue disease, 104
 stimulatory, against TSH receptor, 40
Autoantigen, 400
 B-cell selection by, 393, 400
 pathogenic effects of complexes with, 407, 408, 410
Autograft, 343
Autoimmune disease(s), 366, 367, 386, 390
 factors influencing development of, 398
 males versus females and, 212
 NZBxW F1 hybrid, 397
 organ-specific, 390, 422
 pernicious anemia and, 387, 389
 Sjögren's syndrome and, 388
 systemic, 386, 396, 422
 T-cell mediated hypersensitivity in, 412–414, 416
 of thyroid, 421
 thyrotoxicosis and, 40
 treatment of, 417–420
Autoimmune encephalomyelitis (EAE), 405
Autoimmune hemolytic anemia (AHA), 375, 389, 402
 NZB model of, 395
Autoimmune thyroid disease, 341, 387
Autoimmune thyroiditis, inflammatory infiltrate in, 413
Autoimmunity, 341, 401
 natural, 392
Autoradiography, 123
Autoreactive antibody, 392
Avidity, 101
Azathioprine, 344, 350, 362
AZT, 316, 362

3b, 7
B1 cell, 243
B7, 170
 T-cell ligand binding of, 157
Bacille Calmette-Guérin (BCG), 292, 299
Bacteria
 adherence of, 263
 carbohydrate of, 19, 392
 C3b opsonization of, 8
 damage of, by reactive oxygen intermediates, 4
 defect in killing of, 318
 growing of, within macrophages, 279
 killing of, 1
 opsonization of, 49, 256
 phagocytosis of, 215
 polymorphonuclear neutrophil attack of, by phagocytosis, 16
 (*See also* Extracellular bacteria; Intracellular bacteria)

Bacterial polysaccharides, C-reactive protein and, 11
Bacterial toxin, neutralization of, 49
Bactericidal action, 277
Baculovirus vector, 298
Balb/c mouse, 407
Basedow's disease, 403
Basement membrane, 9
Basophil, 3, 9
Bb, 6, 7
B-blast, 138
   primary, 151
B cell(s) (B lymphocyte), 25, 201
   activation of, 166
      carrier T-cell epitope and, 164
      characteristics of, 155
      cross-linking of B-cell surface receptors and, 166
      in islets of Langerhans, 414
      lipopolysaccharide and, 163
      murine, polyclonal activator of, 163
      resting B cells by T-helpers and, 167
      surface glycoproteins on, 370
      T-cell help for antibody production and, 165
   $CD5^+$, 202
   clonal selection and, 26
   costimulatory signal for, 173
   distinction of, from T cells, 168
   early mature, 64
   expression of IgM and IgD, prior to class switching, 187
   Fcγ receptor on, 218
   germinal center, 181
      features of, 180
   individual, immunoglobulin class switching in, 179
   maturation of, 138
   MHC class II molecules on, 82
   mRNA in, 70
   newly produced, 64
   parent, 27
   production of antibody by, 65, 210
   proliferation, maturation, and secretion of, 28
   responding, autoantigen selection of, 393
   resting, activation of, 167, 173
   selection of, of autoantigen, 400
   specificity of antibody secreted by, 183
   surface receptor on, 53
   virgin, signal transduction after antigen binding and, 67
   (*See also* Primary B-cell deficiency)
B-cell line
   high affinity, 185
   lepromin-specific, 199
B-cell lymphoma, 373
B-cell memory, 138
B-cell ontogeny, 248
B-cell recognition, difference in T cell and, 93
B-cell response, 164
   genuine adaptive, 249
   secondary, 312
B-cell surface receptor
   for antigen, 64–66
   cross-linking of, 166
B-cell tolerance, 247
Beige mouse, 375
Bentonite, 109
β chain, 68, 149, 150, 191
β-pleated sheet, 78
β-turn loop, 47
β-microglobulin, 78
Binding strength of antibody for antigen, 95, 105, 106
Biozzi mouse, 209
Birth, high level of passive immunity at, 246
Blast cell, 136
Blk src kinase, 166
Blood, 3, 23, 135
   antigens in, 134
   cord, 239
   human adult peripheral, 239
   recirculation of lymphocytes and, 147
Blood transfusion, pretreatment with, 352
Body, protection of
   external surfaces of, 1
   mucosal surfaces of, 278
Bone, erosions in, 411
Bone marrow, 142, 225, 226
   reconstitution with, 231, 363
      graft versus host disease and, 353
Bone marrow purging in myeloid leukemias, 383
Bone marrow stem cell, 3, 133
Botryllus schosseri, 249
Bovine serum albumin (BSA), 241
   conjugation of, with dinitrophenol, 172
Bovine spongiform encephalopathy (BSE), 299
Brain, 143
   autoallergic attack on, 390
Brain myelin basic protein, 390
Breast-fed offspring, 285, 368
Brown Norway rat, 415
Bruton's congenital agammaglobulinemia, 305
Burkitt's lymphoma, 367, 376, 382
Burn, 1
BXSB mouse, 415

C1 inhibitor deficiency, 304
C1q molecule, 21
   fixation of, 19
C1qrs molecule, 24
C1r molecule, 21
C1s molecule, 21
C3 convertase, 6, 21, 24, 356, 365
   alternative pathway, 304
C3 molecule, 8, 17, 18
   cleaving of, 6, 21, 24

fixation of, 146
inactive form of, 8
C3a molecule, 6, 8, 17, 24
C3b molecule, 6, 7, 17, 21, 24, 256, 259, 262
    opsonization of bacteria by, 8
    splitting of, 8
C3b receptor, 8, 14
C3bBb C3 convertase, 7
C3bBb molecule, 6, 24
C3d molecule, 8
C3de molecule, 8
C4 molecule, 24
C4b molecule, 24
C4b2b convertase, generation of, 21
C5 convertase, 21, 24
C5 molecule, 24
    splitting of, 7
C5a molecule, 7, 9, 17, 20, 21, 24
    chemotaxis and, 8, 17
C5b molecule, 7, 24
    formation of membrane attack
        complex and, 17
C6 molecule, 24
C7 molecule, 24
C8 molecule, 24, 265
    deficiency in, 304
C9 molecule, 21, 24, 265
Cadaver kidney, 1-year survival rate for, 352
Calcium channel, pre-synaptic, 421
Calcium ion (Ca^{2+}), intracellular, rapid
    mobilization of, 67
Calcium phosphate precipitate, 128
Cancer
    chemically induced, 371
    therapy for, 382, 383
Cancer cells, single clone of, 58
Candida, 37
Capsule of extracellular bacteria, 260
Carbohydrate, 19, 96
    bacterial, 392
Carcinoembryonic antigen (CEA), 385
Carcinoma, 379
    pancreatic, 369
Cardiolipin/β_2-glycoprotein 1 complex, 421
Carrier, 84
Carrier-mediated transport system, 143
Carrier T-cell epitope, 164
Cartilage, erosions in, 411
Cartilage graft, 363
Catalytic antibody, 118
Cationic protein, 5, 279
CBA cell, 241
CD1, 383
CD3, 73, 233, 383
CD4, 67, 69, 154, 158, 169, 311, 399
    depletion of, 322
    lepromin-specific, 199
    numbers of, 314
    profound reduction of, 224

CD4⁺ cell, 82, 198
CD4⁻CD8⁻ cell, 232
CD5, 383
CD5⁺ B cell, 202, 243, 392, 399, 400
CD5⁺B1 subset, 52
CD8 cell, 67, 69, 158, 201, 399
CD8 cytotoxic T cell, 97, 140
CD8 suppressor clone, lepromin-specific, 199
CD8⁺ T cell in gut epithelium, 235
CD28, 157
    ligation of, 170
CD33, 383
CD34, 227
CD40, 167, 173, 181
    ligation of, 173
CD44 molecule, 372
CD45 (leukocyte common antigen), 186, 379
    cell deficient in, 160
    T-cell mutants without, 160
CD45RO, 186, 192
Celiac disease, 405
Cell(s)
    activated, antigen presentation for, 145
    coating of, with specific antibody, 121
    genetic engineering of, 128
    introduction of gene into, 128
    tissue migration of, 149
    virally infected, 20
Cell line, 298
Cell-mediated hypersensitivity, 323
Cell-mediated immunity, 224
    defects in, 385
    macrophage-activating, 288
    protection against intracellular organisms
        and, 39
    T-cell effectors in, 178
Cell surface (molecule), 69, 97, 125
    immunoglobulins on, 67
Cell-surface viral receptor, 32
Cellular basis of antibody production, 27, 28, 34
Cellular recognition molecule, 250
Centroblast, 151
Centrocyte, 139
Cγ 2 domain, 48
C_H sterile transcripts, production of, 182
C_{H1} domain, 57
Chains of T-cell receptor, 68, 69
Chaotropic agent, 120
Chediak-Higashi disease, 303
Cheese washer's disease, 335
Chemotaxis, 9, 26
    C5a and, 8
    for polymorphs, 17, 255
    release of factors involved in, 18, 26
Chemotoxin for polymorphs, 21
Chicken cholera bacillus, 291
Children
    ALL in, 385
    leukemia in, 378

with selective T-cell deficiency, 140
vaccination of, 287
with Wiskott-Aldrich syndrome, 374
Chinese hamster ovary (CHO) cell, 298
Cholera, 291, 292
Chondroitin sulfate, 11
Chromosome, 72
Chromosome 5, 175
Chromosome 8q24, 376
Chromosome 14q32, 376
Chronic granulomatous disease, 303, 318, 340
Chronic infection, site of, 340
Chronic inflammation, granuloma formed by, 258
Chronic lymphocytic leukemia (CLL), 378
Circulating autoantibody, 422
Circulation of two-month-old breast-fed baby, 285
C_L gene, 44
Class I HLA-A and -B molecules, 81
Class switching, 182, 248, 319
B-cell expression before, 187
Classical complement pathway, 17, 21, 24
Cleavage enzyme, 6
Clinical grafting, 352
graft versus host disease and, 353
Clone
proliferation of, 26
during primary immune response, 29
selection of, 26
surface immunoglobulin of, 183
c-myc gene, 188, 376
Codominant expression of MHC genes, 83
Cold hemagglutinin disease, 332
Colicin, 1, 7
Colon, diagnostic marker for tumors of, 385
Colorectal cancer, 369
Combined immunodeficiency, 307
Common acute lymphoblastic leukemia antigen (CALLA), 385
Common acute lymphoblastic leukemia antigen (CALLA)-positive ALL, 378
Complement, 6–8, 21, 24, 38, 259, 277, 339
activation of: by constant region of antibody, 22
first component of, 11, 21
components of, 17, 21, 23
deficiency of, 398
functions of, 26
lysis by, 289
opsonization by, 145
of viruses, 19
reactive lysis and, 333
Complement fixation, 11, 19, 21, 22, 49
by IgG3, 55
Complementarity determining region (CDR), 43
Complete Freund's adjuvant, 296, 390, 396, 412
Confocal microscope, 124, 130
Conjugate of antibody for visualizing tissue antigen, 123

Constant (C) gene segment, 47, 72
activation of complement by, 22
Convertase, 7
Cord blood, 239
Cortical lymphoid follicles, proliferation in, 152
Cortisol, 216
Costimulatory signal, 167
for activation of resting T cells, 170
for B cells, 173
Countercurrent immunoelectrophoresis, 104
Cowpox, 290
vaccination against smallpox with, 31
CR1 complement receptor on phagocytic cells, 262
C-reactive protein, 11, 19
antibacterial action of, 20
Creutzfeldt-Jakob disease (CJD), 299
Cross-linking
of B-cell surface receptors, 166
of DNA, 350
of IgE receptors on mast cells, 326
of immune complexes, 103
of membrane immunoglobulin, 67
Cross-matching for ABO and MHC, 362
Cross-reaction, 394, 401
autoantibody and, 202
idiotype, 206
Cryptic epitope, 368
C-terminal domain, 67
of IgG heavy chain (Cγ3), 48
CTLA-4, 157
Cultured pancreatic insulin-secreting cell, 178
Cyclo-oxygenase pathway, 327
Cyclophosphamide, 350
Cyclosporin, 350, 362
Cysticercosis, ovine, 299
Cytochrome p245 oxidase system, 4
Cytokeratin, 379
Cytokine(s), 26, 174, 175, 177, 190
action of, 191
class switch to IgE production and, 179
imbalance of, 401
mediation of release of acute phase proteins by, 189
production of, protective response and, 317
release of, 93, 126
specific, assay of, 190
T_{h1}-type, 199
T_{h2}-type, 199
type IV hypersensitivity and, 339
upregulation and, 382
Cytokine gene on chromosome 5 in man, 175
Cytokine receptor, 191
Cytomegalovirus infection, 310
Cytoplasmic granule, microbicidal, 3
Cytosolic protein, peptides produced by processing of, 90, 97
Cytotoxic T cell (CTL), 38, 149, 153, 201, 270, 317, 374

Epstein-Barr virus and, 382
steroids and, 350
Cytotoxicity, 93, 126

Decay accelerating factor (DAF), 356, 365
deficiency in, 304
Defensin, 5, 16, 279
Degranulation, 326
of mast cells, 8, 9, 21
Delayed hypersensitivity, 176, 323, 324
skin tests and, 308
δ chain, 68
Denaturation of protein, 85
Der p1 allergen, 328
Development, unregulated, lymphoproliferative disorders and, 376, 378, 379
Dextran, 110, 111
Diabetes, 391
insulin-dependent, 414
Diacylglycerol, 159
Diet, effect of, 215
Differential (alternative) splicing, 65, 187
Differentiation, 377
DiGeorge syndrome, 306, 320
Digestion, 1
Dimerization of IgA, 51, 63
Dinitrophenol (DNP), bovine serum albumin conjugated with, 172
Diphtheria, herd immunity to, 287
Discontinuous antigen epitope, 85
Disease(s)
HLA and, 354, 355
from red cell autoantibodies, 395
world-wide eradication of, 290
Dissociation constant, 88, 110
Disulfide bond, 42, 410
interheavy chain, 57
intra-chain, 47
Diversity (D) gene segment, 44, 45, 59, 60, 72
insertion of nucleotide at N-region of, 75
recombination and, 74
Dizygotic twins, 391
DNA (deoxyribonucleic acid), 125, 139, 397
alkylating and cross-linking of, 350
aminopterin blocks synthesis of, 117
SLE and, 386
DNA antibody in systemic lupus erythematosus (SLE), 104
DNA–anti-DNA immune complex, 409
Domains of immunoglobulins, 47, 48
DQα, 81
DR mismatch, 352
DR2, multiple sclerosis and, 355
DR3, 355
DR4, 355

Earthworm, 249
Effector lymphocyte, 29
Ehrlich, Paul, 34

Electron microscope, 123
Electroporation, 128, 132
Electrostatic interaction, 87
Elephantiasis, 336
Embryo, earliest site of hematopoiesis in, 225
Embryogenesis, 149, 225
Embryonic cells, antigens expressed on, 368
Encapsulated lymph node, 139, 140, 151, 152
Endomyceum, 405
Endoplasmic reticulum, 90
Endosialin, 373
Endosome, 90
Endothelial cell(s), 2, 9, 276
stimulation of, by lipopolysaccharide, 342
Endotoxin, 342
Entamoeba histolytica, 289
Enterocyte, 420
Enterotoxin superantigen, 342
Enzyme(s), 5, 118
cleavage, 6
of complement, 23
Enzyme-linked immunosorbent assay (ELISA), 109
Eosinophil, 3, 20, 329, 334
major basic protein in, 14
Eosinophil chemotactic factor (ECF), 327
Epithelial cell, thymic, 242
Epitope(s), 84, 88, 112, 205, 208
carrier T cell, 164
description of, 94
different, on same antigen, 205
discontinuous antigen, 85
recognition of, by T cells, 116
T cell, 301
Epitope-specific vaccine, 302
Epstein-Barr (EB) virus, 199, 367, 376, 385
vaccine against, 382
Epstein-Barr virus–positive lymphoma, 374
Equilibrium dialysis, 106
Erythema nodosum leprosum, 336
Erythrocyte
sheep, 197
turkey, 107, 111
Estradiol, 357
Estrogenic oral contraceptive, 212
Europium, 109
Exercise, severe, increased susceptibility to infection and, 216
Exogenous antigen, 401
Exon, 65
Exophthalmos, 403
Exotoxin
bacterial, 296
pyrogenic streptococcal, 264
Experimental animal, treatment of, with x-rays, 36
Experimental autoallergic encephalomyelitis, 390
Experimental autoimmune encephalomyelitis (EAE), 416

animals protected against, 419
Experimental autoimmune thyroiditis (EAT), 412, 416
External body surface, defense of, 63
Extracellular bacteria, 260
　　CR1 complement receptors on phagocytic cells and, 262
　　killing of, 260, 277
　　Neisseria infection and, 265
　　neutralization of toxins and, 261
　　optimal killing of, 259
　　pyrogenic streptococcal exotoxins and, 264
　　secretory IgA and, 263
　　(*See also* Bacteria; Intracellular bacteria)
Extracellular fluid, lysozyme in, 10
Extracellular killing, 13, 14
Extracellular matrix, 149, 226, 245
Extracellular organism, 93, 100
Extravillous trophoblast, 356, 365
Eye, anterior chamber of, 143

F1 (A × B) animal, 347
Fab (fragment antigen binding) region, 22, 42, 57, 326
　　function of, 62
$F(ab')_2$, 48, 57, 65
Factor B, 6
　　cleaving of, 24
Factor D, 6, 24
Factor H, 6
Factor I, 6
Familial Mediterranean fever, 380
Farmer's lung, 335, 336
Fas gene, 375
Fc non-antigen binding region, 48
Fc receptor on cell surface, 22
Fc region, 25, 103, 246
Fcα receptor, 51
Fcε receptor, 54, 326
Fcγ receptor, 285
　　on B cells, 218
Fd region, 48
Feedback control for antibodies, 196
Feedback suppression, 214, 385
Female, 212
Fetal αβ T cell, 236
Fetal γδ T-cell receptor cell, 238
Fetal immunology, 357, 358
Fetal mouse spleen, hybridomas established from, 203
Fetus
　　protection of, from maternal transplantation attack, 365
　　recurrent loss of, 402
Fibrin clot, 254
Fibrinogen, 11, 254
Fibroblast, 156, 226, 340
Flow cytofluorimetry, 125
Fluorescein isothiocyanate (FITC), 109

Fluorescence activated cell sorter (FACS), 121, 129
Fluorescent antibody, 130
　　myeloperoxidase and, 131
Fluorescent antigen, 129
Fluorescent conjugate, 123, 124
Follicular dendritic cell, 140, 146, 193
Foreign antigen, major long-term source of, 193
fos/jun protooncogene, 162
Framework region, 76
Free energy change of Ag/Ab interaction, 88
Frustrated phagocytosis, 411
Functional activity, assessment of, 126, 127
Furrier's lung, 335
Fv region, 48
　　antigen-binding single chain, 286

G0 to G1 progression, 188
Ga rheumatoid factor site, 55
γ chain, 68
γ chain gene, 72
γδ T cell, 232
　　with Vγ9, Vγ2 T-cell receptor, 239
γδ T-cell receptor, 71
　　fetal, 238
Gastric acid
　　microorganisms and, 15
　　protection of external body surfaces by, 1
Gastrointestinal cancer, 373
Gene(s)
　　closely linked, 354
　　for immunoglobulin, 44, 45
　　introduction of, into cell, 128
　　selective disruption by, 132
　　upregulation of, by T-cell activation, 188
Gene cluster, 44
　　D region and, 59
Gene pool, 65
Gene shuffling, 248
Genetic engineering, 128
Genetic factor(s), 391
　　high antibody response to antigen and, 210
　　high responder 'Biozzi' mice and, 209
　　poor MHC-linked immune response and, 211
Genitourinary tract, 148
Germinal center, 138, 146, 181, 184
　　development of, 152
　　follicular dendritic cell in, 193
　　mutation of B cells in, 393
　　primary B-blast in, 151
Germinal center B cell, 181
　　features of, 180
Germinal center macrophage, tingible bodies inside, 139
Germline, mutation away from, 393
Giant cell/epithelioid cell, 340
Globular domain, 78, 79
Glomerulonephritis, 366, 390, 397, 406
Glomerulus, 2

Glucocorticoid, 213, 214, 257
  production of, by IL-1, 223
Glutamic acid decarboxylase (GAD), 414
Gluten, 405
Glycoprotein, 23
  surface, 370
Glycosylation, 410
  of recombinant protein, 298
Goiter, 403
Gold particle, 123
Gold-plated sensor chip, 110, 111
Gold salt, 418
Goodpasture's syndrome, 364, 388, 396, 406, 415
gp120 envelope protein, 311, 315, 322
GPGR epitope, 315
Graft between members of same species, 343
Graft rejection, 40
  allogeneic, 362
  first, 344
  hyperacute, 361
  immunological basis of, 343, 344
  nonspecific suppression of, 349
  prevention of, 348, 351
    anti-CD3 and, 349
    cyclophosphamide and, 350
Graft versus host disease, 347
  transplantation of bone marrow and, 353
Gram-negative bacteria, 163, 277
  septic shock associated with, 342
Gram-positive organism, 342
Granular polymorphonuclear cell, 3
Granule(s), 3, 125
  of eosinophil, 3
  peptides in, 5
Granulocyte macrophage-colony stimulating factor (GM-CSF), 175, 176, 200
Granuloma, 258
  chronic, 340
Graves' thyrotoxicosis, 387, 389, 396, 403
Gut
  epithelium of, CD8+ T cells in, 235
  immune defenses in, 420
  microflora of, 1
    colicins and, 7

H-2^a, third party, 351
H-2A, -2E, -2K genes, 77
H-2^b graft, 351
H-2^b skin, 351
H-2^{bxk} graft, 351
H-2^k mouse, 351
Hageman factor, activated, 254
Haplotype, 360
Hapten, 84, 106, 326
Hashimoto's thyroiditis, 332, 386, 387, 396, 403
Hassall's corpuscle, 229
HAT medium, 117
Heart graft, 363

Heavy chain of immunoglobulin, 41, 56, 57, 64
  complementarity determining regions in, 43
  first constant domain of, 22
  V region of, 286
HeLa tumor cell line, 178
Helminth(s)
  potent killers of, 20
  protection against infection from, 281
Hemagglutination, 111
Hemagglutinin, viral, 268
Hematopoiesis, earliest site of, in embryo, 225
Hematopoietic myeloid stem cell, 2
Hemoglobulinuria, paroxysmal nocturnal, 304
Heparin, 327, 339
Hepatitis B antigen, 104
Hepatoma, 385
Herd immunity to diphtheria, 287
Herpes zoster, 367
Heterodimer, 68, 149
  with common β chain, 150
High affinity antibody, 184, 393
High affinity autoantibody, 202, 400
High affinity B-cell clone, 185
High fat diet, 321
High responder Biozzi mouse, 209
High-walled endothelium of post-capillary venule (HEV), 137, 147
Hinge region, 22, 57, 410
Histamine, 18, 251, 327, 329, 339
Histotope, 301
HIV, 310, 313, 367
  binding of, 311
  main site of sequestration of, in lymphoid tissue, 313
HIV antigens, targets for neutralizing antibody and, 315
HLA, 398, 422
  disease and, 354, 355
  unresponsiveness and, 297
HLA-A, 348
HLA-B, 348
HLA-B8, 355, 364
HLA-B27, 355
HLA-C, 348
HLA-D, 348, 352
HLA-DR2, 364
HLA-DR3, 364
HLA-DR4, 364
HLA DR4/DR1 self-antigen, 367
HLA-G, 356, 365
Homing receptor on lymphocyte, 137
Homologous recombination, 132
Horseradish peroxidase, 109
Horseshoe crab, 9
Host immune response, trypanosomes evasion of, 274
Host mRNA, degradation of, 12
Host protein, 282
House dust mite, 328

hsp60, 412
Human
  chromosome 5 of, 175
  IgG crossing placenta of, 49
  major histocompatibility complex in, 345
  peripheral blood of, in adult, 239
  peripheral blood T cell of, 71
Human chorionic gonadotropin (hCG), 357
  vaccines and, 358
Human T-cell lymphotropic virus type 1 (HTLV-1), 310, 368, 382
Humoral autoantibody, pathogenic effects of
  antiphospholipid syndrome and, 402
  celiac disease and, 405
  glomerulonephritis and, 406
  neonatal myasthenia gravis and, 404
  thyrotoxicosis and, 403
Humoral defense, 10–12
H-Y male antigen, 240
Hybrid, 117
Hybridoma(s), 117, 220
  monoclonal antibodies produced by, 203
  T cell, 122
Hydrolysis of phosphatidylinositol diphosphate, 161
Hydrophilic compound, 143
Hydrophobic bonding, 87
Hydrophobic transmembrane sequence, 65
Hydroxyl ion, 4
Hydroxyl radical, 7
5-hydroxytryptamine (5-HT), 339
Hyperacute graft rejection, 361
Hypergammaglobulinemia, 375
Hyper-IgM syndrome, 319
Hyperplasia, reactive B cell, 265
Hypersensitivity
  mediation of, by T cells, 323
  Type I, 327
    Lol pI-V and, 328
    passive cutaneous anaphylaxis and, 325
    Praunitz-Kustner test and, 329
  Type II: ADCC and, 330
    Mycoplasma pneumoniae infection and, 332
  Type III, 331, 333, 335, 366
    dead *Wuchereria bancrofti* and, 336
    Maple bark stripper's disease and, 335
    reactive lysis and, 333
  Type IV, 323, 324, 338
    chronic granuloma and, 340
    major effector molecules involved in, 339
  Type V, 341
Hypervariable region, 76, 221
Hypochlorohydria, 405
Hypothalamus, 223
Hypoxanthine, 117

iC3b, 8
ICAM-1, 149, 253, 382

Idiotype(s), 119, 205, 221, 373
  description of, 46
  epitope-specific vaccines and, 302
  regulatory, on antibodies, 206
Idiotype–anti-idiotype interaction, 220, 243
Idiotype network, 202, 203
  anti-idiotypic immunoglobulins and, 207
  different epitopes on same antigen and, 205
  internal image monoclonal anti-idiotype and, 208
  Jerne nonspecific parallel idiotype set and, 204
  regulatory idiotypes on antibodies and, 206
Immune complex(es), 102
  aggregated, 103
  binding of, 146
  precipitation of, 103
Immune complex glomerulonephritis, 337
Immune complex-induced nephrotic syndrome, 275
Immune recognition, parasites avoiding of, 282
Immune response(s), 213
  control of, 194, 221
  cortisol depression of, 216
  evolution of, 249
  in gut, 420
  intensity of, 217
  stimulation of, 207, 288
  for tumors, 371, 374, 375
Immune surveillance, 366
Immune system, 69
  antigens sequestered from, 143
  nonresponsiveness of, 37
  ontogeny of, 203
  viruses escape of, 280
Immunity
  innate, 1
  for *M. tuberculosis* in mice, 266
  (*See also* Specific type of immunity)
Immunoassay, 190
Immunocompetence, 133, 231, 241
Immunoconglutinin, 409
Immunodeficiency(ies)
  animal model of, 375
  combined, 307
  primary, 317
  recognition of, 308
  secondary, 309, 321
  severe combined (SCID), 307
Immunodiagnosis of solid tumor, 385
Immunofluorescence, 109, 110, 387
Immunogen, 84, 146
Immunogenic tumor, 374
Immunoglobulin (Ig), 69, 372
  allelic forms of, 46
  anti-idiotypic, 207
  classes of, 49–55
  crossing of placenta by, 246
  domains of, 47, 48

with identical peptide structure, 58
peptides chains in, 56
sticky neonatal, 203
structure of, 41–43
surface, 155
of clonal parent, 183
Immunoglobulin A (IgA)
secretions of, 51, 63, 263, 278
by lymphocytes in lamina propria, 141
transport of, 250
Immunoglobulin A (IgA) myeloma, 329
Immunoglobulin-β (Ig-β), 67
Immunoglobulin class switching, 182
in individual B cells, 179
Immunoglobulin constant regions, interaction of, 203
Immunoglobulin D (IgD), 53, 64, 151, 187
Immunoglobulin E (IgE), 54, 108, 272
cytokine involved in class switch for production of, 179
passive cutaneous anaphylaxis and, 325
protection against worm infestations and, 281
in *Trichinella spiralis* infections, 272
Immunoglobulin E (IgE)-mediated anaphylactic reaction, 328
Immunoglobulin E (IgE) receptors, cross-linking of, on mast cells, 326
Immunoglobulin G (IgG), 49, 202, 218, 259, 285, 331
aggregated, binding of, 50
antigen-specific, 196
autoantibodies to, 409
cleavage of, by papain, 57
constant region of, 21
heavy chain of, 48
maternal, transplacental transfer of, 246, 404
in patients with rheumatoid arthritis, 410
production of, 179
Immunoglobulin G3 (IgG3), 55
Immunoglobulin gene (superfamily), 44, 45, 182, 245, 250, 408
rearrangement of, 248
Immunoglobulin idiotype, 221
Immunoglobulin isotype, 61
Immunoglobulin M (IgM), 52, 64, 151, 187, 202
constant region of, C1q and, 21
low affinity, 392
monoclonal, 381
production of, 179
surface, cytoplasmic region of, 66
Immunoglobulin M-α (IgM-α), 67
Immunoglobulin M (IgM) receptor, 244
Immunoglobulin-secreting cell, 142
Immunoglobulin structural variant, 46
Immunoglobulin-type domain, 69, 250
Immunohistochemistry, 123–135
Immunological basis of graft rejection, 343, 344
Immunological contraceptive (vaccine), 357, 358
Immunology
fetal, 357, 358
reproductive, 356
Immunoneuroendocrine network, 223
Immunopathology, 40
Immunosuppression, 350, 374
allogeneic grafts and, 363
Infection, 15, 398
chronic, site of, 340
concentration gradient toward site of, 26
fibrinogen and, 11
IgE levels high in, with *Trichinella spiralis*, 272
increased susceptibility for, stress induced by severe exercise and, 216
inflammation and, 276
from *Mycoplasma pneumoniae*, 332
with *Neisseria*, 265
overwhelming, 16
serum amyloid P component and, 11
susceptibility for, primary immunodeficiency and, 317
T-cell recognition and, 100
vulnerability for, 1
(*See also* Specific type of infection)
Infectious agent
intracellular versus extracellular, 100
other, expression of antigens from, 294
protective antibodies against, 32
Infectious mononucleosis, 376
Infertility, 402
Inflammation, 2, 9, 396
activated Hageman factor and, 254
chronic, granuloma formed by, 258
granuloma formed by chronic inflammation and, 258
histamine and, 251
infection or tissue injury and, 276
inhibition of, 422
initiation of reaction of, 54
opsonization of bacteria and, 256
optimal killing of extracellular bacteria and, 259
platelet activating factor and, 253
polymorph chemotaxis and, 255
P-selectin pairs and, 252
resolution of, 257
(*See also* Acute inflammation)
Inflammatory atrophic gastritis, 387
Inflammatory infiltrate in autoimmune thyroiditis, 413
Influenza, 292
Innate immunity, 1
Inositol triphosphate, 159
Insulin-dependent diabetes mellitus (IDDM), 355, 364, 386, 414, 416, 417
animal model of, 415
Integrin, 149, 245
Intercellular adhesion, 149

Interdigitating dendritic cell, 144, 201
Interferon, 16, 269
   antiviral effects of, 19
   inhibition of viral replication by, 12
   natural killer cells and, 13
   phosphorylation of protein synthesis initiation factor by, 12
Interferon-γ, 93, 176, 200, 219
   killing of intracellular parasites within macrophages and, 39
   synergism of, with TNFβ, 178
Interleukin-1 (IL-1)
   excessive release of, 342
   glucocorticoid production by, 223
   stimulation of glucocorticoid synthesis by, 214
Interleukin-2 (IL-2), 162, 176, 200
   control of expression of, 188
   natural killer cells and, 384
Interleukin-2 (IL-2) receptor, 177, 191
Interleukin-3 (IL-3), 175, 176, 200
Interleukin-4 (IL-4), 175, 179, 200, 219
Interleukin-5 (IL-5), 175, 329
Interleukin-6 (IL-6), 189
   excessive release of, 342
Interleukin-8 (IL-8), 255
Interleukin-10 (IL-10), 219, 356
Intermolecular force, 86, 87
Internal image idiotype, 302
Internal image monoclonal anti-idiotype. 208
Intestinal epithelium, γδ T cells in, 71
Intracellular bacteria, 266, 267
   cell-mediated immunity protects against, 39
   (*See also* Bacteria; Extracellular bacteria)
Intracellular infection, 38, 96
   recognition of, 93
Intracellular killing within polymorphs, 18
Intracellular parasite within macrophage, 39
Intracellular protein, 89, 100
Intrinsic factor (IF), 417
Islets of Langerhans, 386
   β cells in, 414
   inflammatory attack on, 390
Isoelectric focusing, 114
Isograft, 343
Isohemagglutinin, 337
Isotype, 46, 61

Japan, 376, 382
Jarisch-Herxheimer reaction, 337
Jenner, Edward, 31, 291
Jerne nonspecific parallel idiotype set, 204
Joining (J) gene segment, 44, 45, 60, 72, 236
   insertion of nucleotides at N-region of, 75
   recombination and, 74
Jones-Mote sensitivity, 337

κ light chain, 376
Kidney(s)
   cadaver, 1-year survival rate for, 352
   mesangial cells of, 2
Kidney graft, 363
Kinase, very rapid activation of, 166
Kupffer cell, 2

Lambert-Eaton syndrome, 406, 421
Lamina propria, 135
   of intestinal wall, 148
   lymphocytes in, 141
Langerhans' cell, 144, 334
Latex particle, 107
Lazy leukocyte syndrome, 303
Lck kinase, 160
Lepromatous leprosy, 199, 267
   addition of anti-HLA-DQ for, 198
Lepromin-specific B-cell line, 199
Lepromin-specific CD4 T cell, 199
Lepromin-specific CD8 suppressor clone, 199
Leukocyte, isolation of subpopulations of, 121, 122
Leukotriene B4, 9
   from mast cells, 17
LFA-1 molecule, 149, 245
   upregulation of, 253
LFA-3 molecule, 382
Leishmania donovani, 273
Leukemia(s)
   chronic lymphocytic, 378
   myeloid, bone marrow purging in, 383
Leukocyte, 276
Leukocyte adhesion deficiency, 303
Leukocyte common antigen (*see* CD45)
Leukotriene, 327, 339
Lewis Le^a antigen, 373
Ligation
   of CD28, 170
   of CD40, 173
Light, reflected, 110
Light chain of immunoglobulin, 22, 41, 56, 57, 380, 410
   complementarity determining regions in, 43
   surrogate, 244
   V region of, 286
Limiting dilution analysis, 126, 131
Linear antigen peptide in MHC groove, 96
Linkage disequilibrium, 354
Lipopolysaccharide (LPS), 145
   from Gram-negative bacteria, 163
   septic shock and, 342
Liposome transfection, 132
Lipoxygenase pathway, 327
Live attenuated viral vaccine, 295
Liver, 2
   cytokines mediate release of acute phase proteins from, 189
   fetal, 225
Liver DNA gene library, 70
Liver graft, 363

Lock-and-key fit, 34
Lol pI-V allergen, 328
Low affinity FcγRII IgG receptor, 50
Lung, maple bark stripper's disease and, 335
Luteinizing hormone releasing hormone (LHRH), 357
Lymph, 135
    obstruction of flow of, 336
Lymph node(s), 133, 135, 136
    antigen pneumococcus polysaccharide SIII and, 152
    biopsy of, 314
    encapsulated, 139, 140, 151, 152
    entry of lymphocytes into, 137
    macrophages of, 2
    paracortical area of, 140
Lymphatics, 135
    afferent, 137
    efferent, 136
Lymphocyte(s), 25, 133, 136, 140, 147, 194, 217, 340, 413
    activation of, 126
        B7 binding and, 157
        B cells and, 155
        CD4 and, 154
        CD8 and, 153
        early increase in phospholipase Cγ1 activity and, 161
        nuclear AP-1 site and, 162
        proliferation of activated T cells and, 158
        protein tyrosine kinase activity and, 159
        resting naive T cell and, 156
        T-cell mutants lacking CD45 and, 160
    adoptive transfer of acquired immune responsiveness and, 33
    cell surface molecules of, 23
    effector, 29
    entry of, into lymph nodes, 137
    homing receptors on, 137
    increased proliferative response of, for *Mycobacterium leprae,* 198
    intense proliferation of, 390
    in lamina propria, 141
    large granular, 25
    mixing of, of two individuals, 346
    selective loss of suppressors of, 390
    traffic of, between lymphoid tissues, 136, 137
    VLA molecules and, 150
Lymphocyte network, 220
Lymphocyte polyclonal activator, 370
Lymphocyte transfer experiment, 36
Lymphoid cell, 379
    malignant, 377
Lymphoid organ (tissue)
    lymphocytes traffic between, 136, 137, 150
    main site of sequestration of HIV in, 312
    organized, need for, 133, 135, 148
    primary, 133
    recirculation of lymphocytes and, 147
    secondary, 133
    unencapsulated, 148
Lymphokine-activated killer (LAK) cell, 384
Lymphoma(s), 374, 385
    B cell, 373
    Burkitt's, 367, 376, 382
    Epstein-Barr virus–positive, 374
    non-Hodgkin, 379
Lymphoplasmacytoid cell, 381
Lymphoproliferation (*lpr*) gene, 375
Lymphoproliferative disorders, unregulated development and, 376, 378, 379
Lysis, 13
Lysosome, 145
Lysozyme, 18, 19, 27, 75
    splitting of peptidoglycan by, 10

Macrophage(s), 3, 9, 16, 93, 133, 226, 334
    activated, 340
    adherence for, 11
    bacteria growing within, killing of, 279
    description of, 25
    functions of, 145
    germinal center, tingible bodies inside, 139
    granuloma and, 258
    intracellular parasites within, 39
    lymph node medullary, 2
    MHC class II molecules on, 82
    stimulation of, by lipopolysaccharide, 342
Macrophage-activating cell-mediated immunity, 288
Magnetic bead, coating of, with anti-Ig, 121
Major histocompatibility complex (MHC), 67, 69, 77–81, 83, 89, 116, 359, 372
    codominant expression of genes of, 83
    cross-matching for ABO and, 362
    in human, 345
    incompatibility in, 346
        graft versus host disease and, 347
    linear antigen peptide in groove of, 96
    plus processed peptide, 100, 156, 158
        T-cell receptor link for, 169
        T-cell recognition of, 93
    poor immune response linked with, 211
    of vaccine, 301
Major histocompatibility complex (MHC) class I, 38, 97, 199
    gene of, 77
    groove of, 91, 98
    heavy chain of, 78
    plus peptide, 91, 98, 153, 201
Major histocompatibility complex (MHC) class II, 38, 82, 169, 201, 210, 408
    antigen differences between two individuals and, 360
    on antigen-presenting cell, 154
    β chain of, 79
    genes of, 222
        in mouse, 77

plus peptide, 145, 222
thyrocytes expression of, 421
Major histocompatibility complex (MHC) class II haplotype, 346
Major histocompatibility complex (MHC) class III, gene of, 77, 80
Major histocompatibility complex (MHC) groove, 195
Major histocompatibility complex (MHC) haplotype, 116
Malarial circumsporozoite protein, 301
Malignant lymphoid cell, 377
Malnutrition, 309
MALT, 148
Mannose, 11
Mannose binding protein, 11, 19
Mantoux reaction, 337
Maple bark stripper's disease, 335
Marek's disease virus, 382
Mast cell(s), 3, 9, 327, 334, 420
    activation of, 18
    cross-linking of IgE receptors on, 326
    degranulation of, 8, 21
    IgE binding for, 54
    leukotriene B4 from, 17
    products of, 327
Maternal transplantation attack, fetus protected from, 365
Maturation, clonal, 26
Maturation arrest, 377
M cell, 137
Measles, 168, 295
Medawar, Peter, 241
Mediator, production of, 2
Meiotic crossover, 354
Membrane, lysis of, 26
Membrane attack complex (MAC), 7, 21, 24, 38
    C5b initiates formation of, 11
Memory, 33, 37
Memory B cell, 187, 193
Memory cell(s), 192, 193
    activated, 186
    B cells in germinal center and, 181
    secondary immune response and, 29
Mesangial cell, 2, 137
Messenger ribonucleic acid (mRNA)
    in B cells, 70
    reduction in translation of, 12
Metabolic defects, control of, 422
Metastatic spread, 372
Methylcholanthrene (MCA), 371
Microbial antigen, poor skin tests to range of, 308
Microbicidal agent, 3, 303
Microflora of gut
    colicins and, 7
    protection of external body surfaces by, 1
Microorganism(s), 1, 15
    adherence of, 263

C3b opsonization of, 17
carbohydrate of, 19
killed, digestion of, 5
opsonized, binding of, 14
protection against inside cells and, 38
Mimotope, 301
Minor transplantation antigen, 345
Mitomycin C, 346
Mitosis, 126, 346
Mixed connective tissue disease, autoantibodies in, 104
Mixed lymphocyte reaction, 348, 352
MLL gene, 284–287
MLR with homozygous stimulating cells, 348
Mold, susceptibility to infection by, 317
Molecular weight, 115
Monoclonal antibody(ies), 110, 118, 227, 393
    for leukocyte common antigen, 379
    production of, by hybridomas, 203
Monoclonal IgM, 381
Monocyte, 2
Mononuclear phagocyte (system), 2
    steroids and, 350
Monovalent antigen binding fragment, 57
Monozygotic twins, 391
Montague, Lady Wortley, 291
Moth, 298
Mother, transplacental passage from, 202
Mouse, 142
    A strain, 241
    Balb/c, 407
    beige, 375
    bovine serum albumin conjugated with dinitrophenol injected into, 172
    BXSB, 415
    chimeric, 241
    congenital deficiency in C5 and, 247
    deficiency in NK cells in strain of, 375
    fetal $\gamma\delta$ T-cell receptor cells in, 238
    first antigen receptor-bearing cells in thymus of, 234
    $H-2^k$, 351
    high antibody response to antigen in, 210
    high responder Biozzi, 209
    injection of, with very high dose of sheep erythrocytes, 197
    male $H-2^b$ SCID, T cells in, 240
    MHC class II region genes in, 77
    moth-eaten viable (Me^v), 375
    MRL-*lpr/lpr*, 375, 407
    natural antibodies in, 399
    non-obese diabetic (NOD), 390, 397, 415
    nude, 375, 416
    NZBxNZW F1, 415
    SCID, 407
    SJL, 375, 407
    specific immunity to *M. tuberculosis* in, 266
    thymectomized, 202
Mouse mammary tumor virus (MMTV), 382

MRL-*lpr/lpr* mouse, 375, 407
μ heavy chain, 376
Mucosal surfaces of body, protection of, 278
Mucus
    protection of external body surfaces by, 1, 263
    secretion of, microorganisms and, 15
Multiendocrinopathy, 389
Multiple sclerosis, 364, 389
    animal model for, 416
    DR2 risk factor for, 355
Multivalent binding, 50, 51
Mumps, 308
Murine B cell, polyclonal activator of, 163
Murine Mls, 366
Murine stem cell, 227
Mutation(s)
    away from germline, 393
    in NADPH oxidase of phagocytic cells, 318
    in p53 protein, 117
    in tyrosine kinase gene, 305
Mutual interaction, 203
Myasthenia gravis, 341, 355, 364, 386, 421
    neonatal, 404
Mycobacterium, 296, 412
    vaccination against disease from, 288
Mycobacterium leprae, 198
Mycobacterium tuberculosis, 292
    specific immunity for, in mice, 266
Mycoplasma pneumoniae, infection from, 332
Myelin basic protein (MBP), 405, 416
Myeloid leukemia, bone marrow purging in, 383
Myeloma, 58
    amyloid deposits in patients with, 380
    IgA, 329
Myeloperoxidase, 131
    deficiency of, 304
Myrmecia pilosula, 328

NADPH oxidase (system)
    mutations in, of phagocytic cells, 318
    phagocytosis activation of, 131
    polymorph, defects in, 303
Naive histocompatible recipient, 266
Nasopharyngeal carcinoma, 367, 376
Native antigen, 89, 96
Natural antibody, 202, 217, 392
    IgM and, 52
    in mouse, 399
Natural autoimmunity, 392
Natural killer (NK) cell(s), 20, 25, 32, 233, 271, 356, 399
    activated, 384
    interferon, perforin, tumor necrosis factor, and serine proteases and, 13
    mouse strain deficient in, 375
Nature versus nurture, 391
Negative feedback, 214
    on adoptive B-cell responses, 196

Negative regulatory site, 160
Neisseria infection, 265
Neonate, 368
    alloimmune thrombocytopenia in, 332
    myasthenia gravis in, 404
Nephelometry, 103
Nervous system, 69
Neuroendocrine factors, 212
    influence of, 213, 214
Neutralizing antibody, target for, 315
Neutrophil(s), 3, 131
    loss of, 16
    polymorphonuclear, 3
    steroids and, 350
Newborn
    prevention of hemolytic disease of, 196
    rhesus hemolytic disease of, 331
Nitric oxide, 4, 16
Nitroblue tetrazolium test, 131
Nitrocellulose membrane, 114
Nitrogen intermediate, 279
Nitrogen peroxide, 4
Non-Hodgkin lymphoma, 379
Non-obese diabetic (NOD) mouse, 390, 397, 415
Nonspecific parallel set, 203
N-region insertion, 75
Nuclear AP-1 site, 162
Nuclear factor of activated T cell (NF-AT), 188
Nude mouse, 375, 416
NZB model of autoimmune hemolytic anemia, 395
NZBxNZW F1 mouse, 415
NZBxW F1 hybrid, 397

Obese strain chicken, 407, 415
Oncofetal antigen, 368, 385
Oncogenic virus, 367
Ontogeny of immune system, 203
Opsonin, 411
Opsonization, 6, 21, 263, 277
    of bacteria, 49, 256
        by C3b, 8
    with complement, 145
Oral immunity, 294
Organ-specific autoimmune disease, 389, 390, 422
Organism(s)
    killed, vaccines and, 289
    live attenuated, vaccines and, 290–293
Ouchterlony double diffusion method, 111, 112
    spur of, 112
Ovine α-chain, 357
Ovine cysticercosis, 299
Oxygen (O_2), 4, 5
    neutralization of, 14
    (*See also* Reactive oxygen intermediate)

p24 antigen, 314

p39, 167
p53 inhibitor, 373
Pancreatic carcinoma, 369
Pannus, 411
Papain, cleavage of IgG by, 57
Papilloma virus, 382
Paracortical area, 140, 144
Parasitic infection(s)
　avoiding immune recognition in, 282
　defense against, 3
　IgE levels and, 272
　immune complex-induced nephrotic syndrome and, 275
　T_{h1} cells and, 273
　trypanosomes and, 274
Paratope, 84, 208
Paratype, 88
Parietal cell, 387
Paroxysmal nocturnal hemoglobulinuria, 304
Passive cutaneous anaphylaxis (PCA), 325
Passive immunity, 285, 286
　high level of, at birth, 246
Pasteur, 291
Pathogenic effects
　of complexes with autoantigens, 407, 408, 410
　of humoral autoantibody: antiphospholipid syndrome and, 402
　　thyrotoxicosis and, 403
Pemphigus vulgaris, 406
Pepscan technique, 116
Pepsin, 42
　treatment of IgG with, 48
Peptide (chain)
　in basic immunoglobulin molecule, 56
　production of, by processing cytosolic proteins, 97
　promiscuous, 301
Peptide antibiotic, 5
Peptide bond, 300
Peptide hormone from thymus, 228
Peptidoglycan, 342
　splitting of, 10, 19
Perforin, 20
　natural killer cells and, 13
Periarteriolar lymphoid sheath (PALS), 137
Pernicious anemia, 386, 396, 405
　diagnosis of, 387
　Graves' thyrotoxicosis and, 389
　treatment of, 417
Peroxidase, 421
　in eosinophils, 14
Pertussis, 292
Peyer's patch, 133, 141, 148
pFc' region, 48
pH, 303
　affinity chromatography and, 120
　high, 15
Phagocytic cell(s), 26, 148
　CR1 complement receptors on, 262
　mutations in NADPH oxidase of, 318
　professional, 3, 8, 10
Phagocytosis, 2–5, 18, 19, 145, 277
　activation of NADPH oxidase by, 131
　of bacteria, 215
　C3b and, 6
　frustrated, 411
　polymorphonuclear neutrophils attack bacteria by, 16
Phenotype, 360
Phosphatidylinositol diphosphate, 159
　hydrolysis of, 161
Phospholipase Cγ1, 159
　early increase in, 161
Phosphorylation, 67, 159, 166, 188
　activation of membrane components by, 171
Pigeon-fancier's disease, 335, 336
Pinocytosis, 145
Pituitary gland, 223
Placenta, immunoglobulin crossing of, 246
Plaque technique, 127
Plasma cell(s), 51, 140, 148
　production of antibodies by, 25
　secretion by, 27
Platelet, 361, 402
　aggregation of, 342
Platelet-activating factor (PAF), 327, 339
　binding of, 253
Pleiotropism, 174
Pneumococcus polysaccharide SIII antigen, 152
Pneumocystis carinii, 310
Point mutation, 369, 373
Poliomyelitis, 290, 291, 295
Polyclonal activator, 401
　of murine B cell, 163
Polyethylene glycol (PEG), 103
Polyimmunoglobulin receptor, 250
Polymorph(s), 3, 259
　chemotaxis for, 17, 18, 255
　chemotoxin for, 21
　defects in NADPH oxidase system of, 303
　functional activity of, 131
　influx of, 9, 18
　intense infiltration by, 334
　platelet activating factor and, 253
Polymorph defensin, 5
Polymorphonuclear neutrophil, 3, 253, 276
　attack of bacteria by, 16
　proteinase III of, 421
Polyspecific antibody, 392
Positive selection in thymus, 242
Post-yersinia arthritis, 355
Praunitz-Kustner test, 329
Pre–B-cell, 399
Precipitin reaction, 111, 113
Prednisone, 350
Preformed antibody, 361
Primary B-cell deficiency, 305, 306

Primary biliary cirrhosis, 388
Primary immune response, clonal proliferation
    during, 29
Primary immunodeficiency, 317
Primary innate immunity, 303, 304
Primary lymphoid organ, 133
Primary myxedema, 387
Primed animal, 136
Private idiotype, 203
Privileged immunological site, 143
Processed peptide, 89, 90, 97, 100
    binding of, for MHC class I groove, 91
    with MHC class II, 145
Professional antigen-presenting cell, 157
Professional phagocytic cell(s), 3, 8, 16
    lysozyme in granules of, 10
Progesterone, 357, 358
Proliferation, 199
    of activated T cells, 158
    clonal, 26
    in cortical lymphoid follicles, 152
    of T_{h2} cells, 200
Promiscuous peptide, 301
Properdin, 7, 39
Propidium iodide, 125
Prostaglandin, 327, 339, 418
Prostaglandin D_2, 327, 339
Prostaglandin E_2, 257
Proteasome, 75
    cleavage mediated by, 90
Protection, 1
    against microorganisms inside cells, 38
Protein(s)
    cationic, 5
    complement components and, 23
    denaturation of, 85
    detection of, by Western blot, 114
    major basic, 14
    SDS-PAGE separation of, 115
    (*See also* Specific type of protein)
Protein A, 103
Protein-calorie malnutrition, 215, 224
Protein tyrosine kinase activity, 159, 171
Protein vaccine, antibody response for, 300
Proteinase III of polymorphonuclear leukocyte, 421
Proteoglycan, 411
Proteolytic cascade, 23
Proteus mirabilis, 367
Protozoal membrane 14
P-selectin, 251, 252, 276
Psittacosis, 290
Public idiotype, 206
Pulmonary hemorrhage, 406
Purification
    of antigen-specific B cells, 129
    of antigens and antibodies by affinity
        chromatography, 120
Pyrogenic streptococcal exotoxin, 264

Quartan malaria, 275

Rabies, 292
Radiation, 231, 309, 390
    sensitivity of lymphocytes for, 36
Radioactive antigen, 106
Radioactive iodine conjugate, 123
Radioallergosorbent test (RAST), 108
Radioimmunoassay (RIA), 109, 110
Rapamycin, 350
ras gene, 369
Rat(s)
    arthritis induction in, 412
    Brown Norway, 415
Reactive B-cell hyperplasia, 379
Reactive lysis, 333
Reactive oxygen intermediate(s), 5, 7, 14, 279, 303, 318
    bacteria damaged by, 4
    production of, 16
Rearrangement, 72
    Ig gene, 248
    VDJ, 180
Recall antigen, 37
Receptor, cytokines binding of, 191
    (*See also* Specific type of receptor)
Recombinase enzyme, 45, 60, 182
    defect in, 307
Recombination, 155
    homologous, 132
    randon VDJ, 74
Red cell, 304
    (*See also* Erythrocyte)
Red cell autoantibody, 395
Reed-Sternberg cell, 385
Reflected light, 110
Regulatory bypass, 395
Regulatory idiotype on antibody, 206
Rejection of second skin graft, 344
Relative risk, 354
Reproductive immunology, 356
Respiratory burst on activation by eosinophils, 14
Respiratory tract, 148
Resting naive T cell, 156
Reticuloendothelial system (RES), 2
Reverse transcriptase, inhibition of, 316
Rhesus hemolytic disease of newborn, 196, 331
Rheumatoid arthritis, 355, 364, 367, 380, 387, 389, 408, 411
    IgG in patients with, 410
    therapeutic approach in, 418
Rheumatoid factor, 409, 412
Ribonucleic acid (RNA) transcript, primary,
    differential splicing of, 65
Ricin A chain, 349
Rubella, 295
Rye grass pollen, 328
Sabin vaccine, 291, 295

Saliva, amylase of, 1
Salk vaccine, 291
Salmonella-based vaccine, 294
Saponin, 299
Scrapie, 299
Secondary antibody response, 29, 35, 138, 146
Secondary follicle, 312
Secondary immunodeficiency, 309, 321
Secondary lymphoid tissue, 133
Sedimentation coefficient, 106
Sedormid, 332
Selectin, 137
Self antigen, 37, 247, 401
    HLA-DR4/DR1, 367
    sequestered, 366
Self-idiotype, 401
Sensitivity, delayed, 176
Septic shock, association of, with Gram-negative bacteria, 342
Septicemia, 342
Serine, 188
Serine protease(s), 20
    natural killer cells and, 13
Seromucous secretion, IgA in, 51, 63
Serum, detection of antibodies in, 28
Serum amyloid P component, 11
Serum antibody, 338
Serum sickness, 336
Severe combined immunodeficiency (SCID), 307
    mouse with, 407
Sex, 398
Sheep erythrocyte, 197
Sialyl Lewis^x, 252, 276
Side-chain theory of antibody production, 34
Signal transduction, 67
Single chain Fv fragment (scFv), 119
Single radial immunodiffusion (SRI), 113
Sister chromatid, suppression of rearrangement on, 248
SJL mouse, 375, 407
Sjögren's syndrome, diagnosis of, 388
Skin, 1, 238
    anaphylactic reaction in, 325
    γδ T cells in, 71
    injection of tuberculin into, 337
    microorganisms and, 15
Skin cancer, 374
Skin graft, second, rejection of, 344
Skin test(s), 308
    for bacterial antigens, 314
    poor, for range of microbial antigens, 308
Slow reacting substance of anaphylaxis (SRS-A), 327
SM-3 monoclonal antibody, 373
Smallpox, 290
    vaccination against, 31
Sodium cromoglycate, 329
Sodium dodecyl sulfate–polyacrylamide gel electrophoresis (SDS-PAGE), 114, 115
Solid graft, rejection of, 361
Solid tumor, immunodiagnosis of, 385
Soluble molecule, 69
Somatic hypermutation, 75, 76, 183, 185
Spatial complementarity, 86, 95
Species, same, graft between members of, 343
Specificity, 88
    of antibody, 183
        high-affinity B-cell clones and, 185
Spleen, 133–136
    neonatal, 220
Spontaneous systemic autoimmune disease, 397
Spur of Ouchterlony test, 112
Stain with eosin, 3
Staphylococcal protein A, 55
Staphylococcus, 99, 103
Staphylococcus enterotoxin B (SEB), 366
Starch, 1
Stem cell(s), 225–227, 306, 320
    bone marrow, 3
    hemopoietic myeloid, 2
    murine, 227
Stem cell antigen-1 (Sca-1), 227
Stem cell factor (SCF), 226
Steroid, 350
Sticky neonatal immunoglobulin, 203
Stimulation, 207
Streptavidin, 111
Streptococcal exotoxin, 168, 264
Streptococcal infection, 303
Stress
    depression of immune responses by, 213
    effects of, 216
Stromal cell, 226
Subclass, 46
Subgroup, 46
Subtractive hybridization, 70
Subunit vaccine(s), 297
    baculovirus vectors and, 298
    ovine cysticercosis and, 299
    promiscuous short peptides and, 301
    tetanus toxoid and, 296
Superantigen, 92, 264, 301, 366, 400
    of *Staphylococcus aureus*, 99
Superoxide anion, 4
Suppression, 207
    non-specific, 282
Suppressor T cell, 219
    failure of, 394
Surface antigen, 274, 282
Surface glycoprotein, 370
Surface immunoglobulin of B cell, 155
Surface immunoglobulin receptor for antigen, 168
Surface plasmon resonance, 110, 111
Surface receptor, 34
    on B cell, 53
Surrogate light chain, 244

Survival rate for cadaver kidney, 352
Syngeneic transplantable tumor, 371
Synovial lining cell, 411
Synovial tissue, non-lymphoid, 408
Systemic autoimmune disease, 389, 396, 422
　spontaneous, 397
Systemic immunity, 294
Systemic lupus erythematosus (SLE), 104, 212, 366, 386–388, 396, 406, 409
　animal model for, 415
　spontaneous model of, 407

Taenia ovis, 299
Tandem duplication, 354
TAP-1/2 molecule, 90
Target cell(s), 13
　direct lysing of, 25
　membrane of, 13
T cell(s) (T lymphocyte), 26, 133
　activated: proliferation of, 158
　　surface glycoproteins on, 370
　adaptive immune response and, 25
　adult, of strain A, 347
　deficiency of, 308, 317
　direct cytoplasmic effect on, 313
　distinction of, from B cells, 168
　epitopes recognized by, 116
　fusing of, with T-cell tumor cell line, 122
　γδ, 232
　genes upregulated by activation of, 188
　gluten and, 405
　help from, for antibody production, 165
　human peripheral blood, 71
　hypersensitivity mediated by, 323
　immunity to *M. tuberculosis* and, 266
　locally activated, 421
　in male H-2^b SCID mice, 240
　naive, 156, 158, 186
　in paracortical area of lymph nodes, 140
　potent stimulators of, 144
　protection against microorganisms and, 38
　recognition of, 89–96, 324
　　difference in B cell and, 93
　　infected cells by, 100
　　MHC plus processed peptide by, 93
　recognition of antigen by, 165, 210
　regulation of, 197–201
　resting, 156
　　costimulatory signal for activation of, 170
　in thymectomized animal, 231
　(*See also* Specific type of T cell)
T-cell acute lymphoblastic leukemia (T-ALL), 377
T-cell effector in cell-mediated immunity, 178
T-cell epitope, 195, 301
　universal, 301
T-cell gp39 gene, deletions in, 319
T-cell hybridoma, 122
T-cell immunity, failed stimulation of, 297

T-cell immunodeficiency, 293
T-cell leukemia, 382
T-cell mediated hypersensitivity in autoimmune diseases, 412–414, 416
T-cell mitogen, potent, 99
T-cell mutant without CD45, 160
T-cell ontogeny
　allelic exclusion and, 237
　CD8$^+$ T cells and, 235
　fetal αβ T cells and, 236
　fetal γδ T cell receptor cells and, 238
　γδ T cells and, 232, 239
　natural killer cells and, 233
　T cells in male H-2^b SCID mice and, 240
T-cell p39, 173
T-cell (surface) receptor, 68, 70–72, 89, 96, 116, 158, 160, 199, 372
　αα homodimer, 235
　chains of, 69, 72
　gene of, 70, 234, 237, 408
　linking of, to MHC/peptide, 169
　recognition of linear antigen peptide in MHC groove by, 96
　Vγ9, Vγ2, 239
T-cell receptor antigen recognition signal, 73
T-cell receptor Vβ peptide, 419
T-cell response
　genuine adaptive, 249
　poor, 267
T-cell signaling, early event in, 171
T-cell tolerance, 241
T-cell tumor cell line, 122
Terminal deoxynucleotidyl transferase (TdT), 75, 234
Testis, 143
Tetanus, 37, 287, 296
(TG)-A-L antigen, 210
T-helper cell(s), 149, 165, 393, 394, 205
　activation of resting B cells by, 167
　CD4 on, 169
　recognition of MHC class II/antigen peptide by, 222
T-helper (T_{h1}) cell, 200, 201, 219, 420
　cytokine of, 199, 266
　defense against *Leishmania donovani,* 273
　secretion of, 176
T-helper (T_{h2}) cell, 200, 201, 219, 420
　cytokine of, 199
Thiocyanate, 120
Third party H-2^a, 351
Thoracic duct, 135, 147
Three-dimensional image, 124
Threonine, 188
Thrombin, 254, 361
Thrombocytopenia, 332, 402
Thrombosis, 149
Thromboxane, 327
Thymectomy, 202, 231, 417
Thymic medulla, 232

Thymidine, 117
Thymocyte, 242, 421
Thymopoietin, 228
Thymosin, 228
Thymulin, 228
Thymus, 40, 133, 228–231
    first antigen receptor-bearing cells in, in mouse, 234
    defect in development of, 306
    failure of development of, 320
    Hassall's corpuscles in, 229
    positive selection in, 242
    production of peptide hormone by, 228
Thymus-dependent antigen, 164, 172
Thymus-independent natural antibody, 202
Thyroglobulin, 341, 412
Thyroid gland, 386
    autoimmune disease of, 341, 421
    stimulatory autoantibodies against TSH receptor in, 40
Thyroid peroxidase (TPO), 341
Thyroid stimulating hormone (TSH) receptor, 341
Thyroiditis, 390
Thyrotoxicosis, 40, 403
Thyroxine, 341, 417
Time-resolved fluorescence, 109
Tingible body, 139
Tissue(s), 149
    fluids of, 23
    injury of, inflammation and, 276
    localization of antigens in, 130
    visualization of antigen of, 123
Tolerance, 37, 241, 358, 366
    development of, 241
Tolerogen, 37
Tonsil, 133
Toxin(s), 32
    neutralization of, 261
Toxoid, 31, 32, 40
Transcription factor, 188
Transduction, 73
Transfection, 128, 395
Translocation, 376
    recombinase enzymes and, 60
    of V, D, and J Ig gene segments, 45
Transmembrane glycoprotein, 79
Transmembrane ion channel, 7
Transplacental passage from mother, 202, 404
Transplantation, 374
    of bone marrow, graft versus host disease and, 353
Transplantation antigen, 345, 371
Transverse electrophoresis, 114
Trichinella spiralis, 272
Trypanosome, 274
Tuberculin, 308
    injection of, into skin, 337
Tuberculosis, 288, 290, 292
tum⁻ variant, 371
Tumor(s)
    antigens expressed on embryonic cells and, 368
    changes on surface of cells of, 367, 369, 370
    diagnostic marker for, of colon, 385
    immune response for, 371, 374, 475
    metastasis of, 149
    normal immunological control of, 366
    solid, immunodiagnosis of, 385
    strongly immunogenic, 374
    syngeneic transplantable, 371
Tumor antigen, 373
Tumor necrosis factor (TNF), 20, 372
    excessive release of, 342
    MHC class III genes and, 80
    natural killer cells and, 13
Tumor necrosis factor α (TNFα), inhibited activity of, 418
Tumor necrosis factor β (TNFβ), 178
Tumor necrosis factor β receptor, 178
Turkey erythrocyte, 107, 111
Twins, monozygotic versus dizygotic, 391
Type 1 diabetes, 391
Type I hypersensitivity, 327
    Lol pI-V and, 328
    passive cutaneous anaphylaxis and, 325
    Praunitz-Kustner test and, 329
Type II hypersensitivity, 331
    ADCC and, 330
    Mycoplasma pneumoniae infection and, 332
Type III hypersensitivity, 333, 335, 366
    dead *Wuchereria bancrofti* and, 336
    maple bark stripper's disease and, 335
    reactive lysis and, 333
Type IV hypersensitivity, 323, 324, 338
    chronic granuloma and, 340
    major effector molecules involved in, 339
Type V hypersensitivity, 341
Tyrosine, 188
Tyrosine kinase gene, mutation in, 305
Tyrosine kinase membrane receptor, 226

Upregulation
    of adhesion molecules, 251, 276
    cytokines and, 382
    of genes subsequent to T-cell activation, 188
    of LFA-1, 253

V gene, 236
    defective rearrangement of, 211
V6 exon-encoded sequence, 372
Vaccination, 31, 32, 283
    basis for, 35
    herd immunity to diphtheria and, 287
    mycobacterial diseases and, 288
    objective of, 288
    against smallpox, 31
Vaccine(s)

epitope-specific, 302
hCG, 358
immunological contraceptive, 357, 358
killed organisms and, 289
live attenuated organisms and, 290, 295
  BCG and, 292
  chicken cholera bacillus and, 291
  vaccinia virus vectors and, 293
protein, antibody response for, 300
Salmonella-based, 294
subunit, 297
  baculovirus vectors and, 298
  ovine cysticercosis and, 299
  promiscuous short peptides and, 301
  tetanus toxoid and, 296
Vaccinia virus vector, 293
Valency, 106
Van der Waals' force, 87
Variable (V) gene segment, 22, 44, 45, 60, 72, 76
  recombination and, 74
Variable region of antibody, 221, 283
Variolation, 283
Vascular addressin, 137
Vascular endothelium, 251, 372
Vascular permeability, increase in, 18
Vasoactive mediator, 18
Vβ T-cell receptor family, 92
Vesicular stomatitis, 367
Vγ9, Vγ2 T-cell receptor, 239
V_H domain, 57
V_H gene, 44
Viral antigen shift, 268
Viral coat protein, 32
Viral hemagglutinin, 268
Viral infection, 20, 268
  cytotoxic T cells and, 270
  interferons and, 269
  natural killer cells and, 271
Viral mRNA, degradation of, 12
Virus, 16
  complement opsonization of, 19
  escape of immune system by, 280
  infection from, 309
  interferon inhibits intracellular replication of, 19
  oncogenic, 367
  replication of, 316
    inhibition of, 269–271
  susceptibility to infection by, 317
Visna virus, 310
Vitamin B_{12}, 405, 417
V_L gene, 44
VLA molecule, 149, 150
V_{preB}, 244

Waldenström's macroglobulinemia, 381
Wegener's granulomatosis, 388, 402, 406, 421
Western blot, 114
Wheat germ agglutinin, 370
Wiskott-Aldrich syndrome, 374
Worm infestation, 349
  protection against, 281
Wound healing, 149
Wuchereria bancrofti, dead, 336

Xenogeneic tumor, 371
Xenograft, 343
Xenopus, 249
X-ray, 36

Yolk sac, 255

Zymosan, 118

HPA SOUTH EAST
SOUTHAMPTON LABORATORY
LEVEL B, SOUTH LABORATORY BLOCK
SOUTHAMPTON GENERAL HOSPITAL
SOUTHAMPTON SO16 6YD

HPA SOUTH EAST
SOUTHAMPTON LABORATORY
LEVEL B, SOUTH LABORATORY BLOCK
SOUTHAMPTON GENERAL HOSPITAL
SOUTHAMPTON SO16 6YD